Genetics of the Epilepsies

Edited by

Gertrud Beck-Mannagetta V. Elving Anderson
Hermann Doose Dieter Janz

With 36 Figures and 83 Tables

Springer-Verlag
Berlin Heidelberg New York
London Paris Tokyo

Gertrud Beck-Mannagetta, M.D., Assistant Professor of Neurology
Neurologische Abteilung
Universitätsklinikum Rudolf Virchow, Freie Universität Berlin
Spandauer Damm 130, D-1000 Berlin 19

V. Elving Anderson, M.D., Professor of Genetics and Cell Biology
Dight Laboratories
University of Minnesota, 400 Church Street S.E.
Minneapolis, MN 55455, USA

Hermann Doose, M.D., Professor of Pediatrics
Abteilung für Neuropädiatrie
Universität Kiel, Schwanenweg 20, D-2300 Kiel

Dieter Janz, M.D., Professor of Neurology
Neurologische Abteilung
Universitätsklinikum Rudolf Virchow, Freie Universität Berlin
Spandauer Damm 130, D-1000 Berlin 19

ISBN-13: 978-3-642-95555-6 e-ISBN-13: 978-3-642-95553-2
DOI: 10.1007/978-3-642-95553-2

Library of Congress Cataloging-in-Publication Data. Genetics of the epilepsies/edited by Gertrud Beck-Mannagetta ... [et al.]. p. cm. Based on a workshop held in Berlin in Sept. 1986. Includes bibliographies and index. ISBN 0-387-18421-X (U.S.) 1. Epilepsy–Genetic aspects–Congresses. I. Beck-Mannagetta, Gertrud. [DNLM: 1. Epilepsy–familial & genetic–congresses. WL 385 G3283]. RC372.G46 1989 616.8′53042–dc19 DNLM/DLC for Library of Congress 88-38737 CIP

Softcover reprint of the hardcover 1st edition 1989

Typesetting, printing and bookbinding: Brühlsche Universitätsdruckerei, Giessen
2122/3130-543210 – Printed on acid-free paper

List of Contributors

You will find the addresses at the beginning of the respective contribution

Preface

This volume is a second undertaking – following the proceedings of the first workshop published in 1982 under the title *Genetic Basis of the Epilepsies* – to review our current knowledge on the genetics of epilepsies. It also developed from a workshop held in Berlin in September 1986. It contains the papers presented by the speakers, but is revised to incorporate the results of the stimulating discussions.

The main goals of the book are to stimulate communication across traditional disciplinary lines and further collaborative research, as well as to provide pediatricians, neurologists, and geneticists with a basic knowledge for genetic counselling while at the same time putting emphasis on the evidence of heterogeneity in this field. This book contains separate sections on population rates, family studies on selected syndromes, genetics of EEG characteristics, morbidity risk in offspring, and special methods and topics. Among the topics covered are the prospective evaluation of seizure morbidity in offspring of epileptic patients and the relationship of pharmacogenetics to epilepsy, two questions of current interest.

The editors are greatly indebted to Mrs. Ilsebill Brookes, secretary of the Department of Neurology, Universitätsklinikum Rudolf Virchow, Free University Berlin, for her valuable assistance in planning and arranging the workshop. Major funding was provided by the Deutsche Forschungsgemeinschaft; Stiftung Michael; Freie Universität Berlin; Boehringer, Ingelheim; Ciba-Geigy, Frankfurt; Desitin, Hamburg; Hoffmann-La Roche, Grenzach; Knoll, Ludwigshafen; Labaz, Munich; Nordmark, Uetersen; Parke-Davis, Munich, and Schering, Berlin. The editors are indebted to these institutions and firms for their generous support.

The Editors

Contents

Special Topics

Opening Address

D. Janz [1]

A hereditary component has often been discussed as being one of the causes of epilepsy. A historical review of this idea must start with Hippocrates, who emphasized that epilepsy was hereditary in his book "On the Holy Disease". We might consider it paradoxical today that he considered the concept of hereditary disease an argument against a contemporary prejudice – that epilepsy had a supernatural cause. Hippocrates argued that epilepsy was not in any way "holier" than other diseases, because it was hereditary and could even be found in animals. Today, 2500 years later, the generally accepted scientific opinion is that epilepsy is a disease with a hereditary disposition rather than an inevitable "curse."

In my opinion the scientific investigation of the genetic aspects of epilepsy began at the turn of the century with descriptions of familiar progressive myoclonus by Unverricht [15, 16] and Lundborg [12]. Our current understanding rejects the notion that there is a single hereditary epileptic syndrome and distinguishes a group of degenerative diseases sharing clinical, morphological, and biochemical characteristics and having an as yet undefined mode of transmission from the group of epilepsies.

The second phase in the scientific investigation of epilepsy was in the period from 1930 to the middle of the 1950s, when Conrad [1–4], Harvald [7, 8], and Lennox [9–11] performed extensive investigations of twins and descendants of epileptic patients, in some cases with electroencephalography. These studies retained the conceptual framework which divided epilepsy into idiopathic and symptomatic forms.

The current phase of genetic research in epilepsy began in the early 1960s with studies published by J. D. Metrakos and K. Metrakos [13, 14]. Their studies are "modern" in the sense that they used a limited number of well-defined characteristics of epilepsy. Metrakos and Metrakos considered the 2.5–3.5/s spike-wave complex as characteristic of "centrencephalic" epilepsy. Other investigators, including Doose et al. [5, 6], failed to confirm these results, and the concept of centrencephalic epilepsy was less sharply defined than it might have been. The studies published by Metrakos and Metrakos were exemplary, however, since they represented an initial attempt at defining the inheritance of a subgroup of idiopathic epilepsies in order to limit the genetic heterogeneity of these disorders as much as possible.

This goal was formulated and the appropriate assumptions and methods were defined at a workshop held 5 years ago in Minnesota, to which Elving Anderson

[1] Neurologische Abteilung, Universitätsklinikum Rudolf Virchow, Freie Universität Berlin, Spandauer Damm 130, D-1000 Berlin 19.

Genetics of the Epilepsies
Beck-Mannagetta et al. (Eds.)

invited a number of investigators active in clinical and experimental research on the genetic basis of epilepsies. The task of the second workshop was to define the current state of knowledge in this field and to provide for an exchange of information on studies then in progress. In addition, reports on collaborative studies initiated after the first workshop and discussions of the applicability and practicability of special techniques and animal models in investigating the genetic component of epileptic syndromes were planned.

Our task was facilitated by the fact that the International League Against Epilepsy (ILAE) recently established a classification of epileptic syndromes to complement the classification of epileptic seizure types that it presented 10 years ago. The new terminology will contribute to better mutual understanding among researchers and clinicians.

The importance which the ILAE has ascribed to the topic of the workshop is evident in the fact that a Commission on Genetics, Pregnancy, and the Child was created a year ago to deal with questions and problems concerning birth defects and the risk of seizure recurrence.

Before the actual work of the conference begins, I feel obliged to present a personal reminiscence on the human and political relevance of the theme "inheritance and epilepsy". This topic has been virtually tabu in Germany since the end of the Third Reich, because the so-called Law for Prevention of Hereditary Disease prescribed obligatory sterilization in cases of genuine epilepsy. At the time, many – though not all – recognized experts and researchers in the field endorsed this legislation as necessary and effective for the prevention of hereditary disease. This sort of genetic science was both incorrect and inhumane. It was incorrect because many patients were sterilized whose epilepsy would now be considered symptomatic rather than genuine. An example is the condition now termed temporal epilepsy, which was described as typically epileptic at the time. It is inhumane for genetic science to serve political or commercial goals even if the diagnostic criteria are modern.

I may be the senior participant in the workshop and I should claim the prerogative to remind everyone that our knowledge and the results of our research have consequences for which we are responsible. I hope and wish that we remain aware of our responsibility in the course of our work, and would be pleased if we were able to discuss the consequences of our research on genetic counselling during the course of the workshop.

References

1. Conrad K (1935) Erbanlage und Epilepsie. I. Untersuchungen an einer Serie von 253 Zwillingspaaren. Z Neurol 153:271–326
2. Conrad K (1936a) Erbanlage und Epilepsie. II. Ein Beitrag zur Zwillingskasuistik. Die konkordanten Eineiigen. Z Neurol 155:254–297
3. Conrad K (1936b) Erbanlage und Epilepsie. III. Ein Beitrag zur Zwillingskasuistik. Die diskordanten Eineiigen. Z Neurol 155:509–542
4. Conrad K (1937) Erbanlage und Epilepsie. IV. Ergebnisse einer Nachkommenschaftsuntersuchung an Epileptikern (Zur empirischen Erbprognose der Epilepsie). Z Neurol 159:521–581

5. Doose H, Gerken H, Völzke E (1968) Genetics of centrencephalic epilepsy in childhood. Epilepsia 9:107–115
6. Doose H, Gerken H, Horstmann T, Völzke E (1973) Genetic factors in spike-wave absences. Epilepsia 14:57–75
7. Harvald B (1951) On the genetic prognosis of epilepsy. Acta Psychiatr Scand 26:339–352
8. Harvald B (1954) Heredity in epilepsy. An electroencephalographic study of relatives of epileptics. Munksgaard, Copenhagen
9. Lennox WG (1947) The genetics of epilepsy. Am J Psychiatry 103:457–462
10. Lennox WG (1951) The heredity of epilepsy as told by relatives and twins. JAMA 146:529–536
11. Lennox WG, Gibbs EL, Gibbs FA (1939) The inheritance of epilepsy as revealed by the electroencephalograph. JAMA 113:1002–1003
12. Lundborg H (1903) Die progressive Myoklonus-Epilepsie (Unverricht's Myoklonie). Almquist and Wiksel, Uppsala
13. Metrakos JD, Metrakos K (1960) Genetics of convulsive disorders. I. Introduction, problems, methods and baselines. Neurology 10:228–240
14. Metrakos K, Metrakos JD (1961) Genetics of convulsive disorders. II. Genetic and electroencephalographic studies in centrencephalic epilepsy. Neurology 11:474–483
15. Unverricht H (1891) Die Myoklonie. Deuticke, Leipzig
16. Unverricht H (1895) Über familiäre Myoklonie. Dtsch Z Nervenheilkd 7:32–67

Population Rates of Epileptic Seizures and Epileptic Syndromes

Epidemiologic Measurements for the Determination of Genetic Risks

W. A. HAUSER [1] and J. F. ANNEGERS [2]

The tendency for epilepsy to aggregate in families has long been recognized. While it is clear that some diseases for which seizures or epilepsy are included as part of a symptom complex will follow Mendelian patterns of inheritance, in these families the phenotypic expression of the seizures tend to be similar. Such patterns account for only a small proportion of all cases of seizure disorders. For these unique families, linkage studies and gene mapping is appropriate to determine the location of the abnormal gene. In addition, biochemical or other specialized studies are warranted to identify the underlying mechanisms by which seizures occur. Such studies may ultimately lead to clues for all cases of epilepsy.

For the majority of situations in which multiple members of a family have seizures the clinical manifestations are heterogeneous, and the pattern of affected individuals within the family structure does not immediately suggest Mendelian inheritance. In this situation, there are several questions which must be answered to adequately evaluate the significance of an aggregation of cases:

1. Is the frequency of seizures or epilepsy in fact increased above what may be expected by chance? Seizures and epilepsy are relatively common symptoms and the chance occurrence of more than one case in a family – particularly an extended family – is not unusual.
2. Is the frequency of a particular class of seizures increased above that expected? An increase in the frequency of a specific subtype of epilepsy may be informative even in the absence of a general increase in the overall frequency of seizures within a family.
3. When an increase in the frequency of seizures in general or a specific seizure subtype is identified among family members of a patient with epilepsy, does this imply a common environmental exposure or a specific genetic predisposition? While the occurrence of seizure or epilepsy in multiple family members of probands with epilepsy has at times been taken as evidence of a genetic etiology, both epidemiologic techniques and, where appropriate, complex segregation analysis should be utilized to clarify the nature of the familial aggregation. One may look at Kuru and the Parkinson dementia complex on Guam as examples of diseases initially thought to be genetic in which environmental factors have been identified as causal.

[1] G. H. Sergievsky Center, Columbia University, 630 West 168th Street, New York, NY 10032, USA.
[2] School of Public Health, The University of Texas, Houston, TX 77030, USA.

The optimal evaluation of a familial aggregation of seizures or epilepsy requires information about seizures in the proband including characteristics of the ictus, age of onset, and any relevant clinical or laboratory data which may be necessary to allow appropiate categorication of the case. Similar information regarding seizure manifestations and relevant clinical findings are necessary to allow appropriate classification of cases in relatives. The nature of the relationship of the proband to the relative and the age (or age at death), sex, and relationship of all relatives presumed to be unaffected must also be determined. This will allow the calculation of an age (and sex) adjusted risk for seizures or epilepsy in relatives over all and for a specific seizure type. These rates in relatives can then be compared with the population rate to allow determination of changes in risk within the families of interest.

Measures of Disease Frequency for Family Studies

Epidemiologic studies are necessary to address the question of the expected frequency of epilepsy or seizures in the general population. In addition, epidemiologic studies are important for the identification of factors (including genetic predisposition) which may influence these frequencies. There are several basic measures. Each has a different function, and the advantages and disadvantages of each must be understood.

Prevalence is a measure of the proportion of individuals within a population affected with a disease at a particular point (or period) in time. For a disease such as epilepsy, prevalence usually includes individuals who have had a diagnosis of epilepsy who are having seizures at the time of identification or who require limitations of activity because of the disease. The latter group are frequently operationally defined by the need to take anticonvulsant medications. Prevalence is generally useful to those interested in health care policy in order to determine the burden of health care needs for a specific disease. Prevalence studies are usually accomplished through surveys of existing medical records or interviews of selected populations to identify affected individuals at a particular point in time. They have the advantages of being relatively easy to perform, and are inexpensive. Because of the latter, there are many reports in the literature of prevalence in diverse populations. There is a wide variation in the reported prevalence of epilepsy in the literature. Comparison of prevalence rates may allow rough estimates of the relative frequency of an illness across populations which vary by race, geographic area, and socioeconomic status, but these comparisons must be made with caution. In general, variation in rates can be attributed more to differences in the method of case identification than differences associated with biologic factors.

Prevalence rates represent a complex interaction between obvious factors such as incidence, death, or remission of illness. Prevalence may also be affected by less obvious factors such as selective in- or out-migration from a community or a selective drop out from medical care. Prevalence is more a reflection of survivorship and severity or chronicity of illness than of frequency. The study of prevalence cases may give little information regarding etiology. Such cases will more likely provide information on factors related to chronicity or severity.

Studies of the frequency of epilepsy in families should consider the occurrence of seizures or epilepsy in all eligible relatives, and will include an individual as affected whether living or dead and regardless of current seizure status (active or inactive). A first level of elevation in risk can then be determined by comparing the proportion of relatives affected with the epidemiologic data on disease frequency. While some investigators have used prevalence rates to estimate this expected frequency, prevalence rates cannot account for individuals who were affected but, for whatever reason (e.g., death or remission), are no longer considered to have symptoms of the illness. Prevalence is thus not an appropriate basis to determine the expected numbers of cases within families, since its use will underestimate the expected number of cases and thus substantially overestimate the increase in risk within families of probands by a factor of 2 to 4.

Incidence is a measure of the frequency with which new cases of an illness develop in a population. To determine incidence, one ideally should identify individuals at the time of onset of an illness. From a practical standpoint, diseases such as epilepsy are seldom identified at the onset of symptoms, rather after a defined constellation of symptoms and signs have developed which allow a definitive diagnosis to be made. For a patient with epilepsy, the interval between onset of disease and definitive diagnosis is, on the average, 2 years. Incidence cohorts will include a wider spectrum of cases with the illness than prevalence. Only those who die before a diagnosis can be made and those with symptoms which are so mild that they never come to medical attention will be excluded. While this may lead to some underestimation of the incidence of the disease in the population, this underenumeration may have little impact upon comparisons in family studies. For the latter situation, it is unlikely that symptoms will be recognized as such by either the affected individual or his family.

When compared with prevalence, incidence studies not only provide much better information regarding the spectrum of illness, but they are also more likely to provide valid information regarding antecedents of the illness. Individuals are usually identified at an earlier point in the course of their illness, and thus a time closer to the occurrence of presumed etiologic factors. The inclusion of mild cases as well as cases who will die shortly after diagnosis allows evaluation of a wider spectrum of illness severity and the identification of factors which will influence course. From a standpoint of prevention as well as understanding and modifying course of illness, incidence studies provide useful information which may dictate specific action on the part of the clinician.

Unfortunately, incidence studies require ongoing surveillance of a population of adequate size over a period of time sufficiently long to assure stable estimates of frequency. Because of this, they are expensive, and there are few studies available in the literature. Thus far there is little variation in the reported incidence in the several studies and, as with prevalence, these variations are probably related more to the methods of case identification than true differences in disease frequency.

Simplistically, the *cumulative incidence* is the summation of age specific incidence to determine the proportion of the population who has ever been affected with a disease by a specific age. The cumulative incidence determined in the above manner does not take into account mortality. Epidemiologic studies have thus far failed to identify any major increase in mortality for most cases of epilepsy. Thus, for this disease the cumulative incidence at any age will in fact be a close approximation to the prevalence of a history of epilepsy whether current or not. This takes into account the cases which have left the medical system either because of remission of symptoms, use of alternative modes of therapy, and or dissatisfaction with the medical care system.

The appropriate measure for comparing the frequency for families is cumulative incidence. For family studies even the proviso regarding mortality is not important. For the question of risk for epilepsy within families one will determine the current age or age of death of all relatives, and even the adjustment for death is not necessary. One will presumably have information regarding all eligible cases among family members, even those who have expired.

Cumulative Incidence of Seizures and Epilepsy in Rochester, Minnesota

We have determined the cumulative incidence for several classes of seizure disorders for the community of Rochester, Minnesota. These rates can be used to provide estimates for the expected number of cases among family members of probands with epilepsy. They will be valid for communities in which the incidence is similar and if no time trends or cohort effects have occurred which would modify the estimates of incidence of epilepsy.

The lifetime cumulative incidence of epilepsy (recurrent unprovoked seizures) was 4.1% through age 90. The cumulative incidence of epilepsy was higher for males (4.5%) than females (3.8%) (Table 1). It is possible that sex specific rates should be taken into account as well, particularly if one wishes to address differential loading hypotheses or the possible effects of maternal transmission.

For studies of the genetics of epilepsy, one may wish to consider relatives to be affected who have had only a single unprovoked seizure. Such individuals will be better identified at a family level than at a population level and it is likely that our estimates of the incidence of this class of seizure are low. The cumulative incidence for all unprovoked seizures (both single and recurrent) in Rochester, Minnesota, through age 90 was 5.3%. The difference by sex was even greater in this category: 6.1% for males versus 4.8% for females.

Table 1. Cumulative incidence for seizures and epilepsy

Seizure class	Male (%)	Female (%)	Total (%)
Epilepsy	4.5	3.8	4.1
Single unprovoked	1.6	1.0	1.2
Febrile	2.3	2.0	2.2
Acute symptomatic (Nonfebrile)	4.0	2.1	2.9
Any seizure	12.4	8.9	10.4

We have defined *acute symptomatic seizures* as convulsions occurring in the context of a severe systemic metabolic disturbance (i.e., hypocalcemia, uremia) or at the time of an acute insult to the central nervous system (i.e., severe head trauma, cerebrovascular insult). Since the identification of such cases would require review of all cases with the disease in question, it is likely that a considerable underenumeration exists in our estimates of the frequency of occurrence of this class of seizures.

The cumulative incidence for acute symptomatic seizures (excluding febrile seizures) through age 90 was 2.9%. Again, males were more frequently affected than females (4.0% vs 2.1% respectively). This difference in rates by sex may be more a reflection of a higher frequency in males of conditions causing acute symptomatic seizures (head injury, CNS infection, alcoholism) than any selective vulnerability for males to have seizures in association with systemic or brain insults. The cumulative incidence for febrile seizures was 2.2%. This again is higher for males than females (2.3% vs 2.0%).

If the risk for all seizures is considered, over 10% of residents of the community could be expected to experience a seizure of some type at some time. The overall risk is about 50% higher for males than for females. Since there is likely to have been an underenumeration of cases for several classes of seizures included in the above figures, these estimates should be considered conservative.

Age Specific Cumulative Risk

It is obvious that the estimates of cumulative risk will increase with increasing age. This increase is not linear but reflects variation in the age specific incidence of epilepsy. In Rochester, age specific incidence for all epilepsy is high in the first 10 years of life and equally high after age 60. Thus, the slope of the cumulative in-

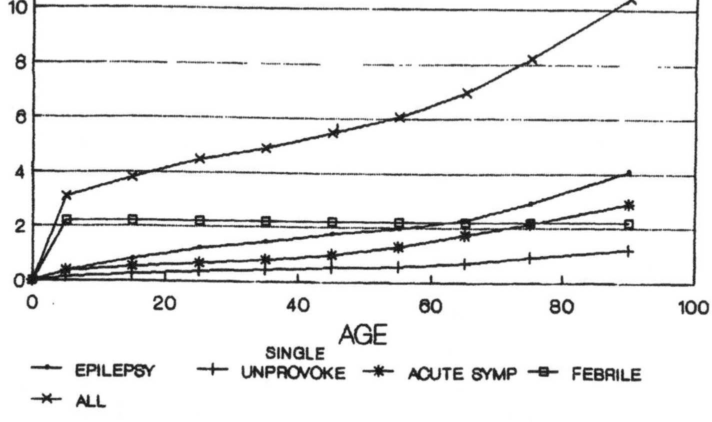

Fig. 1. Cumulative incidence of seizures

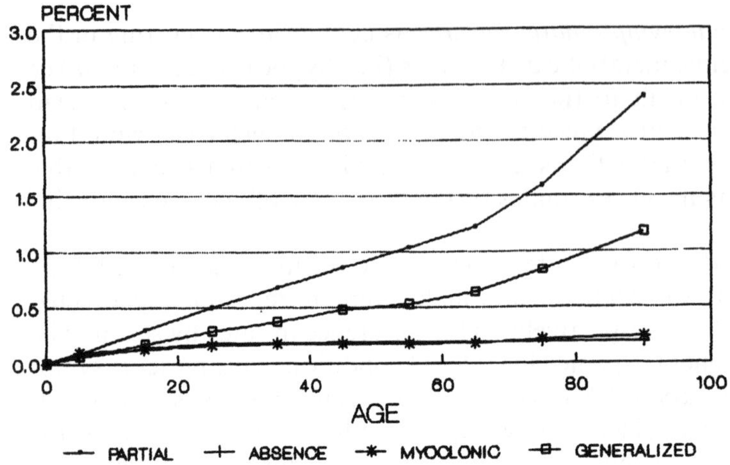

Fig. 2. Cumulative incidence by seizure type

cidence curve is steep in the first 10 years of life, is quite steady for the next 50 years, and then increases again in the elderly (Fig. 1).

In general this same age specific incidence pattern is true for single unprovoked seizures and for acute symptomatic seizures. For febrile seizures, virtually all cases are recognized in the first 5 years of life after which little additional increase is noted. Trends are similar for males and females within each class of seizures although the rate at any age is higher for males.

Seizure Specific Cumulative Incidence

Cases of epilepsy were classified by seizure type based upon clinical description. Age specific incidence for both myoclonic and for absence seizures increased through the second decade after which virtually no further cases are identified (Fig. 2). As with febrile seizures, virtually all ascertainment is completed in childhood and an increase in seizure specific risks can be estimated with certainty for those over age 20. For generalized tonic clonic seizures and for partial seizures, cumulative incidence continues to increase in each subsequent age group through the ninth decade. The increase is linear through the sixth decade (reflecting a constant age specific incidence rate) both for epilepsy manifest by partial and by generalized major motor seizures. The age specific incidence increases for both categories of epilepsy after this age.

Summary

The most appropriate epidemiologic measure of frequency of epilepsy for purposes of genetic studies is cumulative incidence. Use of prevalence will considerably overestimate the risks to relatives for seizures in general and for specific types of epilepsy. While not necessarily applicable to all populations, the data presented in this paper can be used to provide estimates of risks for groups of patients with epilepsy.

Clinical Syndromes of Epilepsy

P. Wolf [1]

The present International Classification of Epilepsies and Epileptic Syndromes [3] makes two major distinctions, one of generalized vs location-related epilepsies and one of idiopathic vs symptomatic epilepsies. Consequently, there are four main groups: idiopathic location-related epilepsies, symptomatic location-related epilepsies, idiopathic generalized epilepsies, and symptomatic generalized epilepsies.

The definition of an epileptic syndrome according to this classification is: "An epileptic disorder characterized by a cluster of signs and symptoms customarily occurring together. The signs and symptoms may be clinical or findings detected by ancillary studies. In contradistinction to a disease, a syndrome does not necessarily have a common etiology and prognosis. Some epileptic syndromes, however, are of great prognostic importance."

While this applies to epileptic syndromes in general, one of the four main categories just mentioned, i.e., symptomatic location-related epilepsies, differs from the three others because it comprises syndromes of great individual variability. As a consequence, a definite subdivision of this syndrome group has not yet been possible. This variability is mainly due to the many possible anatomical sites of epileptic foci, the multiform seizure semiology [2], even at very similar anatomical sites, the various etiologies, and still other factors, not all of which are known.

In contrast, the syndromes of the three other groups are much more uniform. In the case of generalized epilepsies, this uniformity may to some extent be due to the much more global involvement of the brain.

The International Classification defines generalized epileptic syndromes as those involving seizures in which the first clinical changes indicate initial involvement of both brain hemispheres and where the ictal EEG discharge is bilateral from the beginning. Also, the interictal EEG discharge is typically bilateral and symmetric. This contrasts clearly with the location-related epilepsies where the seizures have a focal onset from which the discharge spreads in variable ways and to a variable extent into other parts of the brain. This is typically reflected both in the development of clinical symptoms and signs, and in the ictal EEG. whereas in the interictal EEG there is often some local discharge at the site of the focus.

But in spite of the bilateral involvement of the brain, which is common to all generalized epilepsies, there are different types of generalized seizures, and a variety of syndromes must be distinguished. The differentiations may relate to etiology and pathogenesis, semiology, or both. Etiologically, the distinction be-

[1] Epilepsiezentrum Bethel, Klinik für Anfallskranke – Mara 1, Maraweg 21, D-4800 Bielefeld 13.

Genetics of the Epilepsies
Beck-Mannagetta et al. (Eds.)

tween idiopathic and symptomatic has already been mentioned. Idiopathic diseases are those not preceded or occasioned by another disease, and idiopathic epilepsies are defined as those without known or suspected etiology other than possible hereditary predisposition. Symptomatic epilepsies are those considered to be the consequence of a known or suspected disorder of the central nervous system. In generalized epilepsies, these known or suspected disorders involve, by necessity, important parts of both cerebral hemispheres. They may be specific or nonspecific, the specific comprising rare disorders such as some storage diseases or Lafora's disease. Nonspecific causes seem to be much more common and comprise many different etiologies such as pre- and perinatal brain damage, infectious and metabolic diseases, and malformations. Sometimes they remain unidentified but are inferred from the existence of neurological or mental deficits. Considering that the pathogenesis may be multifactorial, findings indicating symptomatic etiologies do not necessarily exclude that there is a genetic background.

A diagnosis of idiopathic generalized epilepsy usually requires normal findings from clinical and ancillary morphological studies because it is assumed that the seizures, here, are due to an exclusively functional disorder. However, an increase in minimal morphological findings of a dysontogenetic type has recently also been demonstrated in idiopathic generalized epilepsies [10, 11].

In practice, it is not always easy to distinguish an idiopathic generalized epilepsy from one that is symptomatic but of unidentified cause, especially since both epileptic EEG discharges and seizure semiology often do not indicate the etiology.

The phenotype seems to depend much more on the manifestation age of the epilepsy than on etiology. This is a very interesting feature of generalized epilepsies, and seems to suggest that the semiology of generalized seizures depends to some extent on the stage of brain maturation at the age of manifestation.

It will also become apparent, as the major syndromes are described below, that the earlier the age of manifestation, the more variable is the seizure semiology and the higher the probability of a symptomatic etiology.

Syndromes of Generalized Epilepsies in Order of Manifestation

Age

Rare syndromes such as benign familial neonatal convulsions or epilepsy with myoclonic absences [13] are not discussed here. There are six syndromes of some quantitative importance. In all of them genetic components have been demonstrated.

West Syndrome [7] is an epileptic syndrome in infancy with peak manifestation at 3–7 months. It usually consists of a characteristic triad: infantile spasms, arrest of psychomotor development, and the characteristic EEG finding of hypsarrhythmia. The spasms may be flexor, extensor, lightning, or nods, but most commonly they are mixed. Males are more commonly affected, and the prognosis is generally poor. In the great majority of cases, the etiology is symptomatic and mostly nonspecific [12]. The symptomatic group is characterized by the previous existence of signs of brain damage (psychomotor retardation, neurological signs, radiological signs, or other types of seizures) or by a known etiology. There is, however, a small group of idiopathic cases characterized by the absence of previous signs of brain damage and of known etiology. In this subgroup the prognosis is better. However, idiopathic and symptomatic cases can not be differentiated by the seizure semiology.

The Lennox-Gastaut Syndrome [1], or Epilepsy with Myoclonic Astatic Seizures [5], is the generalized epilepsy syndrome of preschool-aged children, manifesting mostly from age 2 to 5 years. A considerable variety of seizures may be seen, such as myoclonic, astatic, myoclonic-astatic, absences, tonic-axial seizures, and tonic-clonic seizures. Focal seizures may also develop. The typical EEG finding is slow spikes and waves. The etiology is nonspecific symptomatic in the majority of cases, but idiopathic cases probably account for 30%–40%. The prognosis is better than in West syndrome but is still quite unfavorable. It seems that, like in West syndrome, the outcome is usually better in idiopathic cases. Tonic-axial seizures seem to be a prominent feature in symptomatic cases but are very rare in the idiopathic variant. Some authors believe that Lennox-Gastaut syndrome and epilepsy with myoclonic astatic seizures should be considered as different syndromes, separated by the absence or presence of this seizure type [13].

The multiplicity of seizure types greatly recedes with increasing manifestation age, and children developing generalized epilepsy during school age usually have absences. These are lapses of consciousness that last for several seconds and may be accompanied by an upward turn of the gaze and head, mild myocloni of the eyeballs and eyelids, and only occasionally other symptoms. In the EEG they are accompanied by spikes and waves with a frequency of 3/s or faster.

Two syndromes of generalized epilepsy are characterized by absences (as the most prominent seizure type).

Pyknolepsy or Childhood Absence Epilepsy [9] is a syndrome that is observed in children of primary school age with peak manifestation at age 6–7 years. In the great majority this is an idiopathic disorder. In contrast to most other epileptic syndromes, there is a predominance of female patients. In this syndrome the absences are very frequent (several to many per day). The response to therapy is good, but in patients who are not sufficiently treated or not treated at all, generalized tonic-clonic seizures may also develop and then the prognosis is less good. Rarely, tonic-clonic seizures manifest before the absences. The development of other seizure types is a rare exception.

Juvenile Absence Epilepsy [14] differs from the previous syndrome in that there is a much lower frequency of absences as they do not occur every day. The manifestation age is considerably later (mean of 14–15 years), and the sex distribution seems to be equal. Association with generalized tonic-clonic seizures is frequent, and they precede the absence manifestations more often than in childhood absence epilepsy. Not infrequently, the patients also have myoclonic seizures. Like pyknolepsy, this is usually an idiopathic disorder, and the response to therapy is usually very good.

Juvenile Myoclonic Epilepsy (Impulsive Petit mal of Janz) [6, 15] usually also starts around puberty. The syndrome is characterized by seizures with bilateral, single or repetitive, arrhythmic, irregular myoclonic jerks, predominantly in the arms. Some patients may suddenly fall from a jerk. No disturbance of consciousness is noticeable. In this syndrome, genetic predisposition is currently being studied in more detail. The sex distribution is equal. Often, there are tonic-clonic seizures and, less often, infrequent absences. All seizure types usually occur shortly after awakening, and are often precipitated by sleep deprivation. Interictal and ictal EEGs have rapid, generalized, often irregular spike waves and poly-spike waves. Frequently, the patients are photosensitive. The response to appropriate antiepileptic drug treatment is very good.

The last of the syndromes of generalized epilepsy to be discussed here is the syndrome in which generalized tonic-clonic or grand mal seizures are the presenting symptom. Grand mal seizures, however, can appear in almost all kinds of epilepsy including location-related epilepsies where a focal onset is typical. But even those that are generalized from the beginning may still form a part of different syndromes.

It has been found, however, that the relationship between grand mal seizures and the various phases of the sleep-waking cycle provides a sensible means of grouping, and the syndrome of idiopathic generalized epilepsy with predominance of tonic-clonic seizures seems indeed to be identified by this procedure.

Epilepsy with Grand mal on Awakening [16] is a syndrome with onset mostly in the second decade of life. The grand mal seizures occur exclusively or predominantly shortly after awakening, regardless of the time of day. There is also a second seizure peak in the evening relaxation period. If there are other seizures, they are mostly absences or myoclonic, as in juvenile myoclonic epilepsy. The seizures may be precipitated by sleep deprivation or other external factors. The EEG shows one of the patterns of idiopathic generalized epilepsy, and there is a significant correlation with photosensitivity.

Location-Related Syndromes

It has been mentioned above that most location-related epilepsies seem to be less consistent in their symptomatology than the generalized epilepsies. This, however, only applies to the symptomatic group which, in location-related epilepsies, is much larger than the idiopathic group. It is even a fairly recent discovery that idiopathic epilepsy may manifest with focal seizures at all. For epilepsy theorists this was rather a surprise because a discharging focus had previously always been expected to be a lesional focus. It is, however, well established now that, in children, discharging foci may be transitory and merely functional. An interesting feature of such epilepsies is that the spike discharge may be recorded from variable loci within a certain region, and that it may even appear alternately in corresponding areas of both hemispheres. The reasons for this are very poorly understood but the very clear age relationship of these disorders suggests again that the state of maturation of the brain or, more precisely, of specific cortical areas may play a role.

There is some indication that other such syndromes may exist [13], but at the moment only one of them is both well established by a significant number of investigations and is of acknowledged quantitative importance.

Benign Childhood Epilepsy with Centro-temporal Spikes [8] is a syndrome of brief, simple, partial, hemifacial motor seizures, frequently having associated somatosensory symptoms, which have a tendency to evolve into generalized tonic-clonic seizures. Both seizure types are often related to sleep. Onset is between 3 and 13 years of age (peak 9–10 years), and recovery is before ages 15–16. Genetic predisposition is frequent and there is male predominance. The EEG has blunt high-voltage centrotemporal spikes, often followed by slow waves that are activated by sleep and tend to spread or shift from side to side. At the moment, this is considered to be the most benign epileptic disorder with a self-limiting development in almost all cases.

Conclusions

To conclude, those epileptic syndromes with only minor interindividual variability seem to belong either to the idiopathic or to the generalized group of epilepsies, or both. Since hereditary factors seem to exist in all idiopathic syndromes, one should assume that their intrasyndromatic homogeneity is due to their common genetic background.

This view, however, is challenged by the observation that, in generalized epilepsies, the most variable etiological factors may produce striking phenocopies of the idiopathic disorders, providing they become manifest at the same age. This seems to indicate that the differences between various idiopathic syndromes are not necessarily due to genetic differences but might be explained by the state of brain maturation at onset, and the manifestation may well depend on external factors, which could accidentally become active at any age.

On the other hand, there is reason to believe that at least one difference between syndromes is genetically determined: Two syndromes of generalized idiopathic epilepsy, juvenile absence epilepsy, and juvenile myoclonic epilepsy have almost identical onset ages. There is also some overlap in that quite a few patients develop both absences and myoclonic seizures. These two seizure types, however, are very different [2]. It has recently been shown that patients with myoclonic seizures have the highest rate of photosensitivity of all idiopathic epilepsies, whereas those with only absences of juvenile manifestation do not show any signs of photosensitivity [17]. Photosensitivity very probably is an inherited feature [4], and its absence or presence in a generalized epilepsy manifesting around puberty seems, thus, to have an important influence on the phenotype.

The various possibilities of interaction between genetic and acquired factors in the configuration of epileptic syndromes remain, in many instances, still open to discussion. We should be prepared to realize more than one of these possibilities in the vast field of epilepsies.

References

1. Beaumanoir A (1985) The Lennox-Gastaut syndrome. In [13], pp 89–99
2. Commission on Classification and Terminology of the International League against Epilepsy (1981) Proposal for revised clinical and electroencephalographic classification of epileptic seizures. Epilepsia 22:489–501
3. Commission on Classification and Terminology of the International League against Epilepsy (1985) Proposal for classification of epilepsies and epileptic syndromes. Epilepsia 26:268–278
4. Doose H (1982) Photosensitivity: genetics and significance in the pathogenesis of epilepsy. In: Anderson VE, Hauser WA, Penry JK, Sing CF (eds) Genetic basis of the epilepsies. Raven, New York, pp 113–121
5. Doose H (1985) Myoclonic astatic epilepsy of early childhood. In [13], pp 78–88
6. Janz D (1985) Epilepsy with impulsive petit mal (juvenile myoclonic epilepsy). Acta Neurol Scand 72:449–459
7. Jeavons PM (1985) West syndrome: infantile spasms. In [13], pp 42–50
8. Lerman P (1985) Benign partial epilepsy with centro-temporal spikes. In [13], pp 150–158
9. Loiseau P (1985) Childhood absence epilepsy. In [13], pp 106–120
10. Meencke HJ, Janz D (1984) Neuropathological findings in primary generalized epilepsy: a study of eight cases. Epilepsia 25:8–21
11. Meencke HJ, Janz D (1985) The significance of microdysgenesia in primary generalized epilepsy: an answer to the considerations of Lyon and Gastaut. Epilepsia 26:368–371
12. Meencke HJ, Gerhard C (1985) Morphological aspects of etiology and the course of infantile spasms. Neuropediatrics 16:59–66
13. Roger J, Dravet C, Bureau M, Dreifuss FE, Wolf P (1985) Epileptic syndromes in infancy, childhood and adolescence. Libbey Eurotext, London Paris
14. Wolf P (1985) Juvenile absence epilepsy. In [13], pp 242–246
15. Wolf P (1985) Juvenile myoclonic epilepsy. In [13], pp 247–258
16. Wolf P (1985) Epilepsy with grand mal on awakening. In [13], pp 259–270
17. Wolf P, Goosses (1986) Relation of photosensitivity to epileptic syndromes. J Neurol Neurosurg Psychiat 49:1386–1391

Epilepsies and Epileptic Syndromes in a Neurological Seizure Clinic

B. SCHMITZ [1] and P. WOLF [2]

Introduction

The International Classification of Epilepsies and Epileptic Syndromes [1] comprises numerous separate entities which are, however, of very unequal quantitative importance. In the previous chapter a number of syndromes were sorted out and described in some detail because they are both frequent and of interest for a discussion on differential genetics in the field of epilepsy.

This will be supplemented now by an overview on the relative frequency of epilepsy syndromes in patients attending an out-patient facility for the special care of epilepsy. It is, however, a clinic for adolescents and adults, and a review from a pediatric clinic would yield quite different figures. In addition, the patients of a seizure clinic are presumably not representative of all people with epilepsy but constitute a selection of difficult and problematic cases. Uncomplicated cases and patients with mild epilepsies are more likely to remain in the care of general practitioners and practising neurologists or are not diagnosed and treated at all [2]. On the other hand, the bias can be assumed to be much smaller than in patient groups of psychiatric or neurosurgical units or of epilepsy centres and institutions.

Material and Methods

The out-patient seizure clinic of the Neurological Department in Berlin Charlottenburg is mainly attended by residents of West Berlin with diagnostic or therapeutic problems. In a retrosepctive study we investigated the files of 699 patients, representing all who were first seen between 1 July 1977 and 1 July 1984, who had at least two consultations and who were given a definite diagnosis of epilepsy (defined by two or more unprovoked unequivocal epileptic seizures). Not considered were 52 patients who probably fulfilled the required criteria but whose files were incomplete.

Of these patients, 303 (43%) were females and 396 (57%) males. Most patients were adults, with a mean age at first visit of 30.8 years (SD 14.4) and a mean age

[1] Neurologische Abteilung, Universitätsklinikum Rudolf Virchow, Freie Universität Berlin, Spandauer Damm 130, D-1000 Berlin 19.
[2] Epilepsiezentrum Bethel, Klinik für Anfallskranke – Mara 1, Maraweg 21, D-4800 Bielefeld 13.

Genetics of the Epilepsies
Beck-Mannagetta et al. (Eds.)

at onset of epilepsy of 19.5 years (SD 14.9), the latter figure being significantly lower in females at 17.7 (SD 13.7) years versus 21 years (SD 15.7) in males (Wilcoxon–Mann-Whitney summed ranks test: $p<0.05$).

Patients were classified according to the ICEES. In the group of symptomatic location-related epilepsies the ICEES leaves open several possibilities of subclassification. We classified according to seizure types and their probable anatomical implications. We differentiated patients with simple focal seizures (either evolving

Table 1. Symptoms indicating temporal-limbic involvement

Auditory
Olfactory
Gustatory
Autonomic
Dysmnesic (e. g. "deja vu")
Ideational (e. g. "forced thinking", "dreamy state")
Complex hallucinations

Table 2. Epilepsies and epileptic syndromes: sex distribution and ages at manifestation

	n	%	Ratio males:females	Mean age at manifestation
Location-related epilepsies				
With simple focal seizures, without temporal-limbic involvement	60	8.6	1.3	31.9
With simple focal seizures, with temporal-limbic involvement	54	7.7	1.8	29.6
With complex focal seizures	157	22.5	1.0**	21.7
Only focal seizures evolving to GTC seizures	39	5.6	2.0	26.7
Idiopathic generalized epilepsies				
Pyknolepsy	52	7.5	1.0	8.8*
Juvenile absence epilepsy	56	8.0	1.7	14.3*
Juvenile myoclonic epilepsy	64	9.2	1.1	15.3*
Epilepsy with grand mal on awakening	32	4.6	1.9	17.3*
Other	68	9.8	1.3	25.0*
Generalized idiopathic or symptomatic epilepsies				
West syndrome	1	0.1	0.1	2.0
Lennox-Gastaut syndrome	12	1.7	1.4	6.3
Epilepsies undetermined whether focal or generalized				
With both generalized and focal seizures	52	7.5	1.5	11.4
Without unequivocal generalized or focal features	50	7.2	1.5	20.6

Asterisks refer to figures significantly different from the total of all other syndromes in the same group: * $p<0.05$ (Wilcoxon-Mann-Whitney summed ranks test); ** $p<0.01$ (χ^2 test).

Table 3. Relation between epileptic syndromes and etiological factors

		Familial predisposition		Febrile convulsions		Pre- or perinatal		Exogenous factors	
	n	*n*	%	*n*	%	*n*	%	*n*	%
Localization-related epilepsies									
With simple focal seizures, without temporal-limbic involvement	60	4	7	2	3	8	13	36	60*
With simple focal seizures, with temporal-limbic involvement	54	6	11	4	7	12	22	25	46
With complex focal seizures	157	16	10	21	13*	44	28	42	27**
Only focal seizures evolving to GT seizures	39	2	5	–		15	38	18	46
Idiopathic generalized epilepsies									
Pyknolepsy	52	14	27	3	6	9	17	–	
Juvenile absence epilepsy	56	10	18	6	11	11	20	1	2
Juvenile myoclonic epilepsy	64	24	38*	6	9	3	5	–	
Epilepsy with grand mal on awakening	32	7	22	2	6	7	22	–	
Others	68	7	10	–		4	6	4	6
Generalized idiopathic or symptomatic epilepsies									
West syndrome	1	–			–	1	100	–	
Lennox-Gastaut syndrome	12	5	41	2	16	6	50	1	8
Epilepsies undetermined whether focal or generalized									
With both generalized and focal seizures	52	3	6	10	20	16	31	10	19
Without unequivocal generalized or focal features	50	3	6	5	10	20	40	14	28

Asterisks refer to figures significantly different from the total of all other syndromes in the same group: * $p<0.01$ (χ^2 test); ** $p<0.001$ (χ^2 test).

or not evolving to generalized tonic clonic (GTC) seizures) from those with complex focal seizures (either evolving or not evolving to GTC seizures, either accompanied or not accompanied by simple focal seizures) and patients with exclusively focal seizures evolving to GTC seizures. Those characterized by simple focal seizures were subdivided into those with seizure symptoms indicating involvement of the temporal lobe and limbic system and those without such symptoms. The symptoms taken as indicating temporal-limbic involvement are listed in Table 1.

In the case of syndrome overlap in generalized epilepsies, i.e. when a patient could be classified in different ways, he was classified according to the diagnosis at the onset of the epileptic disorder. Febrile convulsions, however, were not considered as diagnosis at onset but as a precursor syndrome relevant for pathogenesis.

Results and Discussion

The distribution of patients on the various syndromes is given in Table 2, together with sex distribution and ages at manifestation. Males predominate in focal epilepsies, with the exception of epilepsy with complex focal seizures. Idiopathic generalized epilepsies are distributed about evenly in both sexes. Manifestation ages of generalized idiopathic epilepsies are significantly different from each other, indicating their specificity compared with focal epileptic syndromes.

All information on etiological and pathogenetic factors were extracted from patient-files. The results are given in Table 3. Familial predisposition was defined by the occurrence of at least one non-febrile epileptic seizure in relatives of first-to third-degree.

Although one must bear in mind that this is a retrospective study in which information has not been gathered in a systematic and unbiased way, it is interesting to note that familial predisposition seems increased in juvenile myoclonic epilepsy. Febrile convulsions seem to predispose to epilepsy with complex focal seizures, whereas other relationships may have remained undetected due to small numbers. Exogenous factors are correlated with epilepsy with simple focal seizures not involving the limbic-temporal system and are rarely described in epilepsy with complex focal seizures.

References

1. Commission on Classification and Terminology of the International League Against Epilepsy (1985) Proposal for classification of epilepsies and epileptic syndromes. Epilepsia 26(3):268–278
2. Zielinsky JJ (1974) Epidemiology and medical social problems of epilepsy in Warsaw (Final report on research program NO. 19-P-58325-F-01. DHEW, Social and Rehabilitation Services). Washington DC:US Government Printing Office

Family Studies on Selected Syndromes

Genetic Analysis of Febrile Convulsions: Twin and Family Studies

T. Tsuboi [1]

Introduction

Febrile convulsions (FC) have been studied from many aspects, including the genetic and the environmental [3, 5, 7–12]. Despite the intensive investigations, however, our knowledge regarding the role of inheritance remains inadequate. This discrepancy may be due to a number of factors, including definitions of FC, sampling methods, investigated areas, and ages of children investigated [9–12]. Children with FC usually have a good prognosis, and generally only severely sick children visit our clinic, reporting prolonged convulsions or many recurrences. Therefore to avoid a bias in sampling one must investigate an unselected population of children with FC, and preferably over a large area [10]. The present study concerned itself with genetic aspects of all children with FC in the geographically delimited Fuchu area of Tokyo and at our outpatient clinic.

Subjects

Population Sample. A clinical, electroencephalographic, epidemiologic, and genetic study was conducted on all 3-year-old children in Fuchu City (population, 182000 on January 1, 1975) who came to the Fuchu Health Center for regular health examination during the 5 years and 8 months from 1 November 1974 to 30 June 1980; the total number of children examined was 17044. Patients' age upon examination was 37 months. All children with a history of seizures of any type received neurologic and EEG examinations at least twice, at ages 3 and 4 years. The investigation covered 95% of the total population of 3-year-olds in the Fuchu area. From the overall population, randomly selected same-age children (10%) with no seizure history were used as controls.

Clinic Sample. A total of 1689 patients with FC and under 5 years of age at the first clinic visit were examined on numerous aspects. FC was defined in this study as a seizure that occurred soon after the onset of elevated temperature (at least 38 °C), excepting brain infections and gross structural abnormality of the brain [10].

[1] Tokyo Islands Health Center, 3-5-1 Marunouchi, Chiyoda-ku, Tokyo 100, Japan.

Genetics of the Epilepsies
Beck-Mannagetta et al. (Eds.)

Results and Discussion

Twin Study

Twenty children (16 pairs) with FC by age 3 among 96 pairs of twins (10.4%) were examined. The incidence of FC did not differ between males (11%, 11/103) and females (10%, 9/89), and the incidence was only slightly higher in twins than in singletons (8.9% for males, 7.5% for females, [10]). One monozygotic twin male had his first FC at age 7. Schiøttz-Christensen [8] reported the incidence of FC among twins as 2.6% (85/1631 twin pairs), which is nearly the same as that in European population [7]. Thus no correlation between FC and twinning seems to exist.

The pairwise concordance rate of FC was 44% (4/9 pairs) in monozygotic (MZ) and 14% (1/7 pairs) in dizygotic (DZ) twins in the population study. In the clinic sample the concordance rates were 67% (6/9 pairs) and 14% (1/7 pairs), respectively (Table 1). The pairwise concordance rate was higher in MZ than in DZ twins (56% [10/18] versus 14% [2/14], p[Fisher] = 0.020). The concordance rate in MZ twins differed between clinic and population samples (67%, 44%) but was the same in DZ twins (14%). The probandwise concordance rate was 71% (20/28) for MZ and 25% (4/16) for DZ twins.

A higher concordance rate of FC in MZ than in DZ twins was previously indicated in two studies [7, 8], and the difference in the pooled data was statistically significant (32/64 or 50% in MZ, 13/97 or 13% in DZ twins; $\chi^2 = 25.646$, $p < 0.001$). The rate in DZ twins was nearly the same in all studies and was similar to the morbidity risk in siblings (14%, 16/114 [8], 18%, 20/111 [7]). The rate in the present study however was lower (14%, but 25% for probands) than the morbidity in siblings of FC children in the population sample (25%, 342/1373) and in the clinic sample (25%, 429/1687) (see Table 6). DZ twins might be expected to have a greater morbidity than siblings because they share a more similar environment than do siblings both during intrauterine life and in early childhood. Our results did not support an important role for environmental causes of FC.

A previous study [8] reported larger concordance rate in MZ female than in MZ male twins: 7.1% (1/14) versus 58% (7/12). Results in the present study, how-

Table 1. Pairwise concordance rate for febrile convulsions in twins

Authors	Monozygotic twins		Dizygotic twins	
	No. of pairs	Concordance (%)	No. of pairs	Concordance (%)
Schiøttz-Christensen [8]	27	9[a] (33.3)	37	5 (13.5)
Lennox-Buchthal [7]	19	13 (68.4)	46	6 (13.0)
Present study				
Population-based	9	4 (44.4)	7	1 (14.3)
Clinic-based	9	6 (66.7)	7	1 (14.3)
Total	64	32 (50.0)	97	13 (13.4)

[a] Includes one pair of FC proband with epilepsy co-twin.

Table 2. Intrapair similarity of clinical symptoms in 12 concordant twin pairs (10 monozygotic, 2 dizygotic)

Probands			Co-twins (a)	Co-twins (b)	Similarity %	Correlation in twins	Correlation in sib-pairs: Clinic	Correlation in sib-pairs: Population
Age at onset in months	≦19	(a)	12	3	75	+0.466	+0.320	+0.201
	≧20	(b)	3	6		($p<0.05$)	($p<0.001$)	($p<0.001$)
Fever (°C)	<39	(a)	14	1	92	+0.822	+0.313	+0.299
	≧39	(b)	1	8		($p<0.001$)	($p<0.001$)	($p<0.001$)
Number of recurrences	1	(a)	4	4	67	+0.250		
	2 (+)	(b)	4	12		(ns)		
Exogenous factors	present	(a)	22		100	+1.00	+0.293	+0.158
	absent	(b)		2		($p<0.001$)	($p<0.001$)	($p<0.01$)
Recurrence after age 3	yes	(a)	6	6	50	+0.407		
	no	(b)	6	6		($p<0.05$)		
Development of non-febrile seizure	yes	(a)	2	2	83	+0.554		
	no	(b)	2	18		($p<0.01$)		
Duration of seizure (min)	1–4	(a)	12	1	88	+0.749		
	5 or more	(b)	2	9		($p<0.001$)		
First EEG	par	(a)	8	2	83	+0.657		
	np	(b)	2	12		($p<0.001$)		
	basic	(a)	2	1	92	+0.619	+0.471	
	nb	(b)	1	20		($p<0.001$)	($p<0.001$)	
Repeated EEG	par	(a)	10	1	92	+0.832	+0.327	
	np	(b)	1	12		($p<0.001$)	($p<0.001$)	
	basic	(a)	4	1	92	+0.791	+0.557	
	nb	(b)	1	18		($p<0.001$)	($p<0.001$)	

par, paroxysmal abnormality comprising spike and/or spike-and-wave, excluding small or positive spikes; np, no paroxysmal abnormality; basic, background abnormality comprising higher amount of slow waves for his age and/or significant hemispheric difference; nb, no background abnormality.

ever, showed the reverse relationship: 73% (8/11) for males versus 29% (2/7) for females. This difference cannot be explained.

The ratio of concordance rates in MZ and DZ twins is 2 for autosomal-dominant, 4 for autosomal-recessive, and more than 4 for multifactorial inheritance [6]. The ratio of 5.2 (68%/13%) which was observed in one study [7] can be interpreted as indicating that multifactorial inheritance is likely. However, the ratio in the present study was 3.9 and that in another study [8] was 2.5; these findings lead to no definite conclusions. The ratio was larger in our clinic study than in our population study (4.7, 67%/14% versus 3.1, 44%/14%); a similar difference is evident between the findings of a Copenhagen population study [8] and those of a clinic study [7]. This depends on the selection of subjects. In addition to the high concordance rate of FC in MZ twins, similar clinical symptoms – including age at onset of FC, clinical course, and EEG findings – were found. In discordant MZ twins similar EEG findings were observed in all eight pairs.

Intrapair distributions of clinical symptoms in 12 concordant twin pairs (10 MZ, 2 DZ) are indicated in Table 2. Similarity was defined as the clinical symptoms of the same category for each item in the proband and his co-twin. Similarity varied from 50% to 100%, and the correlation between categories varied from +0.327 to +1.00 (Table 2). All ten items except number of FC recurrences showed statistically significant positive correlations. Clinical symptoms with high intrapair positive correlations were: exogenous factors (e.g. perinatal complications such as caesarean section, neonatal asphyxia, jaundice, low birth weight, toxemia during pregnancy), degree of fever (38 °–39 °C, the lowest temperature was registered if FC recurred), abnormality in EEG findings, development of nonfebrile seizure, duration of seizure (shorter than 5 minutes; the longest duration was registered if FC recurred), and age at onset (8–19 months).

In clinical symptoms with high intrapair correlation in twins (+0.75–+1.00), such as exogenous factors, degree of fever, and EEG, heredity can be regarded as playing an important role. A positive correlation was also observed in FC siblings, bot not as strong as in the case of twin pairs. The correlation coefficient for each symptom in unrelated FC children is, as would be expected, nearly zero. The results therefore suggest an important hereditary role in these four items.

Analysis of Siblings

The population sample included 1406 FC children (8.2%), 311 of whom had FC siblings (total 330). These siblings were analyzed in the same way as those in the first section. As shown in Table 3, correlation analyses showed positive relationships among the following factors: age at onset of FC, exogenous factors, and degree of fever. No significant correlation however was found regarding other symptoms. Also these results indicate that heredity plays a role in these factors.

The majority of FC probands in the population study have not yet been treated. The number of recurrences may therefore be considered to indicate the degree of severity of the illness. Frequency of FC recurrences in the probands varied positively with incidence of the disease in siblings of FC probands (Table 4).

Morbidity Risks Among Near Relatives

Morbidity risks among near relatives were 12% in parents, 25% in siblings, 4% in aunts and uncles, and 4% in cousins (Table 5). The difference of incidence between parents and siblings was large ($p<0.001$), as was that between first- and second-degree relatives ($p<0.001$). Differences, on the other hand, between second- and third-degree relatives, between fathers and mothers, and between brothers and sisters were small.

Morbidity risks of FC among near relatives previously reported were 33%–68% in MZ twins, 13%–14% in DZ twins, 8%–32% in siblings and parents, and 8.4% in offspring [5]. The risk was decreased in more distant relatives, such as

Table 3. Similarity in clinical symptoms in FC probands and affected siblings (Population study)

Clinical symptoms in probands			Affected siblings Number	Clinical symptoms (a)	Clinical symptoms (b)	Similarity %	Correlation coefficient
Age at onset of FC (months)	≦19	(a)	173	116	57	62	+0.201
	≧20	(b)	105	49	56		($p<0.01$)
Exogenous factors	Present	(a)	96	19	77	71	+0.158
	Absent	(b)	234	20	214		($p<0.01$)
Fever	<39° C	(a)	108	64	44	65	+0.299
	≧39° C	(b)	95	28	67		($p<0.001$)
Number of recurrence	1	(a)	157	73	84	51	+0.046
	2 (+)	(b)	172	76	96		(ns)
Recurrence after age 3	Yes	(a)	47	7	40	79	+0.049
	No	(b)	276	29	247		(ns)
Development of non-febrile seizure	Yes	(a)	9	0	9	95	−0.025
	No	(b)	321	7	314		(ns)
EEG findings	par	(a)	88	35	53	36	+0.035
	np	(b)	120	48	72		(ns)
	basic	(a)	35	2	33	76	+0.010
	nb	(b)	173	16	157		(ns)

Siblings with inadequate information are excluded.
par: paroxysmal abnormality; basic, background abnormality; np; no paroxysmal abnormality; nb: no background abnormality.

Table 4. Number of recurrence in FC probands and cumulative incidence among siblings

Authors	*N*	i	*N*	i	*N*	i	*N*	i
Fukuyama et al. [4] clinic study	1–4	18%			5–9	21%	10+	29%
Tsuboi [9] population study	1–3	19%			4+	40%		
Tsuboi [11] population study	1	22%	2–4	26%	5+	35%		
Tsuboi [11] clinic study	1	21%	2–4	21%	5+	28%		

N, Number of FC recurrence in probands; i, cumulative incidence FC among siblings.

aunts and uncles (4%, second-degree relatives) and cousins (4%, third-degree relatives). The figure thus declined with increasing remoteness of the blood relationship, particularly from first- to second-degree relatives. These results seem to indicate a hereditary role in the pathogenesis of FC. The rather low figures observed in second- and third-degree relatives and in parents of controls may be attributed to underreporting (difficulty in recall, not being asked for information on the ill-

Table 5. Incidence of FC among near relatives of FC children and controls

Near relatives	Population study						Clinic study		
	FC probands			Controls			FC patients		
	N	*n*	%	*N*	*n*	%	*N*	*n*	%
Father	1259	153	12.2	1324	19	1.4	1652	301	18.2
Mother	1259	144	11.4	1324	30	2.3	1652	262	15.9
Brothers	685	186	27.2	729	78	10.7	853	205	24.0
Sisters	688	156	22.7	652	57	8.7	855	188	22.0
Paternal									
Uncles	2444	86	3.5	2565	15	0.6	2709	154	5.7
Aunts	2220	58	2.6	2260	13	0.6	2460	104	4.2
Male cousins	3069	125	4.1	3402	57	1.7	3834	165	4.3
Female cousins	3020	98	3.2	3188	27	0.8	3807	137	3.6
Maternal									
Uncles	2103	118	5.6	2311	53	2.3	2346	184	7.8
Aunts	2189	98	4.5	2150	41	1.9	2394	158	6.6
Male cousins	2668	125	4.5	2783	83	3.0	3105	191	6.2
Female cousins	2653	116	4.4	2695	61	2.3	3047	131	4.3

N, Total number of relatives; *n*, number of children with seizure.

ness, etc.). However, morbidity risk in siblings of controls (9.8%) was quite similar to the incidence in the general population in the Fuchu area and on Miyake Island (8.2%–10.0% [10]).

Racial and geographical variations in different areas – for example, a high incidence of FC in Japan and the Mariana Islands compared with that in USA and Europe – have been described and discussed elsewhere [10]. Unfortunately there is as yet no explanation for such variations. The ratio of morbidity risk in siblings to that in the general population (p) stands at 7 in USA (14%/2% [5]) and in Denmark (14%/2% [8]) and at 3 in Japan (this study, 25%/8.2%). Expressed theoretically this ratio equals $1/\sqrt{p}$. The analysis shows that polygenic inheritance is most likely as elaborated by Edwards [1].

Segregation Analysis

Morbidity risks among near relatives in the population study were compared if a parent had had FC, or if neither parent had suffered from FC (Table 6). In each case morbidity risks were highest if both parents had had FC, intermediate if one parent had suffered from FC, and lowest if neither parent had had FC. If one parent had had FC, a higher risk was observed in siblings (37% : 21%, $p<0.001$) and in aunts and uncles (6.7% : 3.1%, $p<0.001$); however, the difference in cousins was small (4.5% : 3.9%, ns) compared with that in healthy parents.

Segregation analysis on controls in the present study showed results similar to those in FC probands: the risk in siblings was 51% if one parent had suffered from FC versus 8.3% if neither parent had had the illness, 5.7% versus 1.2% in aunts and uncles, and 5.4% versus 1.8% in cousins ($p<0.001$, in each case).

Table 6. Incidence of febrile convulsions among siblings, uncles and aunts, and cousins of FC probands and controls

Near relatives	Parents	Population study						Clinic study		
		FC probands ($n=1272$)			Controls ($n=1323$)			FC patients ($n=1652$)		
		N	n	%	N	n	%	N	n	%
Siblings	Both with FC	26[a]	12	46.2	–	–	–	37[f]	18	48.6
	One with FC	288[b]	107	37.2	49[d]	25	51.0	452[g]	153	33.8
	father only	145	46	31.7	18	12	60.0	233	79	33.9
	mother only	143	61	42.7	31	13	41.9	219	74	33.8
	Neither	1059[c]	223	21.1	1332[e]	110	8.3	1198[h]	258	21.5
	Total	1373	342	24.9	1381	135	9.8	1687	429	25.4
Uncles, aunts	Both with FC	161	21	13.0	–	–	–	311	27	8.7
	One with FC	1759	118	6.7	316	18	5.7	2505	224	8.9
	Neither	7036	221	3.1	8970	104	1.2	7093	349	4.9
	Total	8956	360	4.0	9286	122	1.3	9909	600	6.1
Cousins	Both with FC	182	10	5.5	–	–	–	431	16	3.7
	One with FC	2176	99	4.5	351	19	5.4	3269	181	5.5
	Neither	9052	355	3.9	11717	209	1.8	10093	427	4.2
	Total	11410	464	4.1	12068	228	1.9	13793	624	4.5

N, number of relatives; n, number of affected relatives.
Number of probands: [a] 25, [b] 278, [c] 994, [d] 50, [e] 1274, [f] 53, [g] 455, [h] 1144.

The segregation ratio in siblings of 1652 FC patients at the clinic was similar: 49% if both parents had had the illness, 34% if one parent had suffered from FC, and 22% if neither parent had had FC. Corresponding morbidity risks were 67%, 23%, and 18% [4] and 56%, 22%, and 5.5% [5], respectively. Morbidity risks in siblings were higher when the mother had had the illness than when the father had had FC (43% : 32%, ns). Other researchers have observed similar results (31.5% : 19% [4], however Frantzen et al. [3] reported an inverse relationship (5.3% : 12%). The observed maternal preponderance may be partly due to the fact that personal interviews were more frequently conducted with mothers than with fathers. However, the present author also personally interviewed grandmothers on both sides, inquiring as to FC in childhood among the parents.

Heritability

Heritability of the predisposition to FC was calculated at 77%, using incidence in the general population and that in siblings of FC children (0.0825 and 0.249, respectively, in the Fuchu study) [2]. Heritability was 71% for males and 78% for females. This figure for heritability indicates that many FC children have developed the disease on a hereditary basis, while others have been influenced by the environment and in still others both inheritance and environment have played a role.

Summary

Thirty-two twin pairs and 673 siblings with febrile convulsions (FC) were studied. Of the 32 twin pairs 16 pairs were from the population study and 16 from the clinic study. Our findings were as follows:

1. Incidence of FC in twins by age 3 in the population study was 11% for males (11/103) and 10% for females (9/89); both rates were slightly higher than those in singletons (8.9%, 7.5%, respectively).
2. The pairwise concordance rate for FC was 56% (10/18 pairs) in monozygotic (MZ) and 14% (2/14 pairs) in dizygotic (DZ) twins ($p<0.05$). The proband-wise concordance rates were 71% (20/28) and 25% (4/16), respectively ($p<0.01$).
3. Intrapair similarity of clinical symptoms in concordant twin pairs (10 MZ, 2 DZ) was greater than that in sibling pairs. A positive, statistically significant correlation was found on ten items; five of these – exogenous factors, degree of fever, duration of seizure, paroxysmal and background EEG abnormality – showed a correlation coefficient of $+0.75-+1.00$, suggesting an important hereditary role.
4. No evident cause was detected in eight discordant MZ co-twins, and many dissimilar symptoms were observed in two concordant DZ twins.

In the population study 1406 children with FC were examined (8.2% of a total 17044). There were 330 sibling pairs affected by FC. A high positive correlation in some clinical symptoms – in particular, age at onset of FC ($r=+0.201$, $p<0.01$), exogenous factors ($r=+0.158$, $p<0.01$), and degree of fever ($r=+0.299$, $p<0.001$) were indicated.

Morbidity risk was higher in first-degree relatives than in second- or third-degree relatives in the population study. The differences found were in the following (descending) order: siblings (24.9%), parents (11.8%), uncles (4.5%), aunts (3.5%), male cousins (4.4%), female cousins (3.8%). Heritability was estimated to be 77%.

References

1. Edwards JH (1960) The simulation of Mendelism. Acta Genet Stat Med 10:63–70
2. Falconer DS (1965) The inheritance of liability to certain diseases, estimated from the incidence among relatives. Ann Hum Genet 29:51–76
3. Frantzen E, Lennox-Buchthal M, Nygaard A, Stene J (1970) A genetic study of febrile convulsions. Neurology 20:909–917
4. Fukuyama Y, Kagawa K, Tanaka K (1979) A genetic study of febrile convulsions. Eur Neurol 18:166–182
5. Hauser WA, Annegers JF, Anderson VE, Kurland LT (1985) The risk of seizure disorders among relatives of children with febrile convulsions. Neurology 35:1268–1273
6. Krüger J (1973) Zur Unterscheidung zwischen multifaktoriellen Erbgang mit Schwellenwerteffekt und einfachem diallen Erbgang. Humangenetik 17:181–252
7. Lennox-Buchthal MA (1973) Febrile convulsions: a reappraisal. Elsevier, New York
8. Schiøttz-Christensen E (1972) Genetic factors in febrile convulsions: an investigation of 64 same-sexed twin pairs. Acta Neurol Scand 48:538–546
9. Tsuboi T (1977) Genetic aspects of febrile convulsions. Hum Genet 38:169–173
10. Tsuboi T (1984) Epidemiology of febrile and afebrile convulsions in children in Japan. Neurology (Cleveland) 34:175–181
11. Tsuboi T (1986) Seizures of childhood: a population-based and clinic-based study. Acta Neurol Scand 71, suppl 110:237
12. Tsuboi T (1987) Genetic aspects of febrile convulsions: twin and family study. Hum Genet 75:7–14

Absences

H. Doose [1] and W. K. Baier [1]

Introduction

Absences have been regarded as an epileptic symptom since the 18th century [25]. Their clear delineation, however, was achieved later, by means of the EEG. The long and controversial discussion about their nature was settled when Jung [16] recorded spike-wave patterns accompanying pyknoleptic seizures. Moreover, catamnestic studies found that pyknoleptic absences of school-age children often later evolved into an epilepsy with grand mal attacks [13, 23].

Electroclinical Definition and Nosology

In the proposal for the revised Classification of Epileptic Seizures of the International League Against Epilepsy [3], *absence* is clearly defined and delineated from other types of absence-like seizures, i.e., the so-called atypical absences. Although this definition considers all essential features of absences, it certainly simplifies the biological spectrum of age-dependent, primarily generalized minor seizures, which includes many intermediate types.

The symptomatological term *absence* does not reflect a nosological entity because absences occur in entirely different clinical types of epilepsy [8]. These are:

1. *Absence epilepsy of early childhood*
   The onset is before the age of 5 years.
   Boys are more often affected than girls.
   At the onset, or later, generalized tonic-clonic and/or myoclonic-astatic seizures may occur.
   The EEG shows irregular 2–3/s spikes and waves and theta rhythms.
   The prognosis is often unfavorable.
2. *Absence epilepsy of later childhood*
   The onset is between 5 and 7 years, absences are the presenting symptom.
   Girls are more often affected than boys.
   Generalized tonic-clonic seizures may arise between 9 and 15 years (usually as "grand mal on awakening").
   The EEG shows regular 3/s spikes and waves.

[1] Abteilung für Neuropädiatrie, Universität Kiel, Schwanenweg 20, D-2300 Kiel.

Genetics of the Epilepsies
Beck-Mannagetta et al. (Eds.)

3. *Juvenile absence epilepsy*
   The onset is between 9 and 12 years of age.
   There is no sex preponderance.
   Frequently, generalized tonic-clonic seizures occur at the onset or later.
   The EEG shows faster spike and polyspike wave patterns.
   The prognosis is doubtful.

Furthermore, absences may occur in epilepsies whose nuclear symptomatology is primarily generalized tonic-clonic or myoclonic.

This classification of epilepsies with absences describes nosological clusters rather than strictly delineated disease entities. In practice, many epilepsies with absences belong to intermediate types.

Genetics

The genetic determination of absence epilepsy was recognized by Lennox [17] in 1951. In identical twins, he found concordance rates of 84% with respect to the 3/s spike-wave pattern, and of 75% with respect to petit mal seizures, as opposed to a concordance of 0% in dizygotic twins [18].

In their fundamental study of the genetics of centrencephalic epilepsy, Metrakos and Metrakos [20, 21] concluded that there is an autosomal dominant "centrencephalic EEG trait." The penetrance of this assumed EEG trait was thought to be age dependent. This study, however, did not consider absence epilepsies in detail.

According to the family studies of Matthes and Weber [19], only 9% of the siblings of patients with absences manifested spikes and waves (12% of the sisters, 9% of the brothers). Detailed data about age distributions, sex of the index cases, or familial incidences of seizures, however, were not communicated in this paper. Doose et al. [10] investigated the families of 239 patients with different types of epilepsies with absences. This study supported multifactorial inheritance, but not an autosomal dominant trait.

Valid information about the risk of seizures among the offspring of absence patients is not yet available. This has, above all, methodological reasons. For the most parts, only those patients have been available who were still under treatment as adults. Hence these samples are biased selections of unfavorable cases and neglect those patients whose disease was definitely controlled in childhood. Beck-Mannagetta and Janz [5] reported on such a selected sample. They found a general risk in the offspring of 6%–8%. In children of epileptic fathers it was 7.7%, in children of epileptic mothers 6.6%, i.e., there were no so-called maternal effects. In not detecting these, this study contradicts others, which reported an increased risk of seizures in the offspring of females as compared to males affected with primary generalized epilepsy [1, 2, 6, 12, 14, 15, 27, 28]. These other studies, however, did not consider absence epilepsy separately from other types of epilepsy. Apart from biases of case ascertainment, efforts to explain these maternal effects have to consider models including a polygenic threshold, maternal transmission in the stricter sense, or both [22]. Up to now, these efforts have not yet produced conclusive results.

Proceeding from earlier studies [9, 10], Doose and Baier [11] analyzed the findings from 400 families with children having different types of primarily generalized minor seizures. In addition to absences (361 cases), this study also included epilepsies with myoclonic-astatic seizures, which often cannot be strictly delineated from the early infantile type of absence epilepsy (see above). The results of this study clearly supported genetic heterogeneity of epilepsies with primarily generalized minor seizures.

It has been shown that the type of familial loading with seizures is related to the type of epilepsy in the index case and his or her siblings, i.e., the different clinical courses are due to qualitatively different genetic dispositions. Doose and Baier [11] studied 87 families of index cases whose parental generation reported seizures. Since the data pertaining to the parental generation were mostly anamnestic, it did not seem sensible to try an exact nosological classification of seizures and epilepsies in the ancestry. It was, however, possible to ascertain the age at onset, which is more readily accessible than details about seizure symptomatology. Therefore, a differentiation was made between seizures in family members that manifested before ("A seizures") and after ("B seizures") the 5th birthday. Febrile convulsions, by definition arising before the age of 5 years, were designated as A seizures. A familial history of A seizures was related to an early onset of epilepsy in the index cases (Fig. 1). These children contracted predominantly convulsive, i.e., febrile or afebrile tonic-clonic or myoclonic-astatic seizures, and less often absences. In the case of a familial history of B seizures the onset occurred later and "nonconvulsive" epilepsies with absences prevailed. In addition to pro-

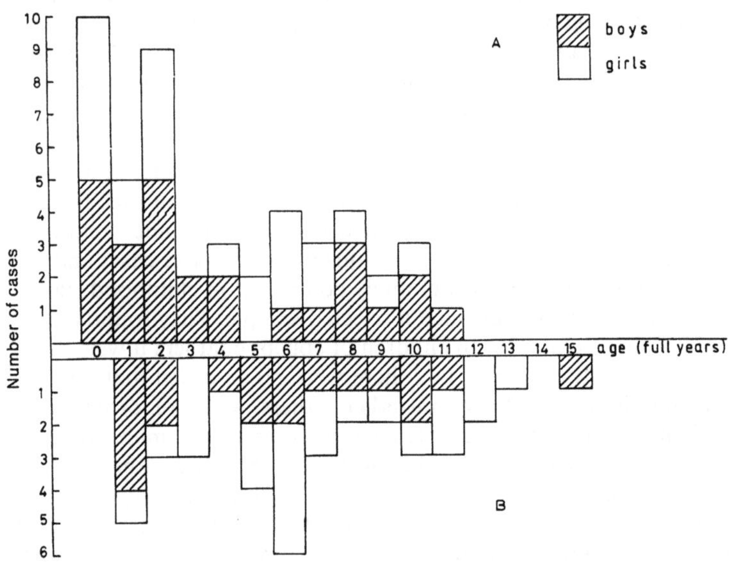

Fig. 1. Age at onset in 87 probands with a seizure-affected parental generation. *Top,* probands with an A affected parental generation; *bottom,* probands with a B loaded ancestry

bands, these differences in symptomatology were also observed in probands' siblings.

This, in itself rather homogeneous, behavior of A and B impact and seizures demonstrates that A and B symptomatology are not just different expressions of a continuous genetic liability on the quantitative scale. They are, most likely, qualitatively different phenomena, resulting from qualitatively different sets of genetic factors. Each of these sets of factors is maximally penetrant during certain maturational phases, the A set during the first years of life, and the B set beyond the 5th year. This, however, does not allow the conclusion that A and B factors were mutually exclusive alternatives, with A and B epilepsies as their clinical expressions. Indeed, there are two different distributions, each probably bimodal, but there is a considerable overlap. As discussed in detail elsewhere [11], the data allow the conclusion that the A factor is largely identical to the genetic background of febrile convulsions. This is supported not only by the clinical correlations, but also by the segregation of seizure types and EEG pathology in the families. These results explain many observations about the pathogenetic relations between febrile convulsions and epilepsy in the stricter sense (for literature, see [11], such as the increased incidence of febrile convulsions in the offspring of mothers affected with epilepsy [2, 4, 27, 28], and especially in children of parents with generalized seizures [4]. Certainly, the widespread disposition to febrile convulsions will be expressed in only a part of its carriers. In the present context this means that even if A seizures could not be ascertained in the parental generation, the A factor may well have influenced the offspring, i.e., the index cases and their siblings.

In the series from Doose and Baier [11], the siblings' risk of seizures of any type was 10%. Twenty-five percent of the affected siblings manifested absences. A pathological EEG occurred in 38% of the siblings and 17% of the total population studied showed spikes and waves during rest or hyperventilation. Only the latter group exhibited a remarkably increased risk of seizures. Other factors influencing the siblings' risk factor were studied in detail. It was demonstrated that the presence or absence of seizures in the parental generation as a whole had no significant effect on the risk of siblings of probands (Table 1).

Family history, if not further specified, does not seem to be a very useful criterion in estimating the siblings' risk. However, a propensity in the maternal gen-

Table 1. Sibling risk in parentally affected and nonaffected families [11]

Probands		Parents affected	Siblings	
N	Sex		*N*	Seizures (%)
44	Male	Yes	76	7
43	Female	Yes	87	14
87	Male + female	Yes	163	10
159	Male	No	249	8
124	Female	No	190	8
283	Male + female	No	439	8

Table 2. Seizure risk in siblings of probands with affected paternal (pat.) or maternal (mat.) parental generation [11]

Probands	Affected parental line[a]	Type	Siblings		
N			*N*	Seizures	%
21	Pat.	A	32	1	3
18	Pat.	B	34	1*	3
39	Pat.	A or B	66	2*	3
27	Mat.	A	46	5	11
21	Mat.	B	51	10*	20
48	Mat.	A or B	97	15*	16

[a] Parent or parent's sibs.
* $p<5\%$.

Table 3. Parents' EEG and siblings' seizure risk in families with affected and unaffected parental generation [11]

Parents' EEG		Parental generation affected	Families	Siblings	
Father	Mother		*N*	*N*	Seizures (%)
0/normal	Path.	No	18	28	21
0/normal	Path.	Yes	14	33	21
0/normal	Normal	No	48	93	2
0/normal	Normal	Yes	9	12	8

0, not investigated.

eration (mothers or mothers' siblings) with A or B seizures resulted in a distinctly higher risk in the probands' siblings than did an affected paternal generation (Table 2). If mothers showed an abnormal EEG (spikes and waves, photosensitivity, dysrhythmia), the risk in the probands' siblings was distinctly increased (Table 3). Whether the parental generation manifested seizures or not was insignificant in this context. Therefore, the maternal EEG is, of the parameters tested in this study, the best predictor of siblings' risk. This is explained by the fact that only 26% of the mothers with an abnormal EEG manifested seizures. So, the EEG is more appropriate for detecting seizure liabilities which remained subthreshold in the mothers. In this series, the risk in siblings is almost exclusively explained by a clinically or subclinically affected maternal generation. This result cannot be due to an – probably often important – paternal underreporting, because these data were collected from those families in which the maternal or paternal generation did report seizures.

Moreover, the results suggested that the different age-dependent epileptic syndromes with generalized minor seizures are genetically distinct from each other. This evaluation was based on three subsamples:

Group I: epilepsies with myoclonic-astatic seizures and absences (in part also with generalized tonic-clonic attacks); onset between 0 and 4 years ($N=107$, 73 boys, 34 girls).

Table 4. Incidence and ratio of A and B seizures in relatives of groups I, II, and III [11]

	N	A seizures %	B seizures %	Ratio A/B
Siblings				
Group I	160	11.9	3.1	3.84
II	183	7.1	3.3	2.15
III	172	6.4	3.5	1.83
Parents				
Group I	202	3.0	2.0	1.50
II	192	2.1	6.3	0.33
III	167	1.2	6.6	0.18

Table 5. Distribution of A seizures in the families of group I and of B seizures in the families of group II. Relatives of female/relatives of male probands

	Group I (73 ♂, 34 ♀) A seizures		Group II (23 ♂, 70 ♀) B seizures	
	Ratio	%	Ratio	%
Brothers	18.2/14.3	1.3	3.6/ 0	~
Sisters	11.1/ 7.3	1.5	5.1/ 0	~
Fathers	5.9/ 4.6	1.3	2.9/ 3.5	0.8
Mothers	0/ 1.5	0	7.4/12.1	0.6

Group II: epilepsies with absences at the onset; starting between 5 and 7 years (N=103, 33 boys, 70 girls).

Group III: epilepsies with absences (and, in part, additional generalized tonic-clonic seizures), onset beyond the 7th year of age (N=69, 42 boys, 27 girls).

The results of these comparative evaluations can be summarized as follows. Whereas the total incidences of seizures in the families of the three groups were nearly equal, the types of seizures exhibited the following differences (Table 4): In the parents of myoclonic-astatic probands (group I) an impact with A seizures prevailed, while the parents of absence patients (groups II and III) were more often affected with B seizures. In the case of siblings and of parents of group I to group III, the ratio of A to B seizures continously decreases. Among the affected siblings of group I, only 13%, but 25% and 29%, respectively, of groups II and III manifested absences.

Depending on the sex of the index cases, A and B seizures showed different familial distributions (Table 5). In epilepsies of early onset (group I), affecting boys more often than girls (73/34), A seizures are more frequent in the families of female index cases than in the families of male index cases. Mothers of female probands, however, are slightly less frequently affected than mothers of male probands. Different results were obtained in group II, comprising absence epilepsies with an onset between 5 and 7 years of age. Here, girls are much more often affected than boys (70/33). Concerning B seizures, the pattern is partially reversed compared to group I A seizures. The risk of B seizures is lower than that of A seizure for the relatives (both mothers and fathers) of female probands. However, the risk is higher for relatives (brothers and sisters) of female probands than of male probands. Finally, male relatives in group I are more often affected with A seizures, whereas B seizures prevail in female relatives in group II. Although, according to conventional statistics, the distributions are not significantly different, they are partially in aligment with certain model assumptions. According to Cloninger [7], the distribution of A and B seizures follows the isocorrelational multifactorial model in many aspects. The isocorrelational multifactorial model assumes a higher threshold for clinical disorder in the less frequently affected sex, and thus predicts that relatives of patients of the less frequently affected sex have a higher mean liability, and are more often affected, than relatives of patients of the more frequently affected sex.

These interpretations are certainly preliminary because the familial patterns are not fully compatible with those predicted under this model. Certainly, the A and B factors do not reflect simple genetic conditions. Moreover, they are not mutually exclusive alternatives, with "A" and "B epilepsies" as their clinical expressions. As demonstrated above, it is sensible to assume an occasional interaction of the A and B sets of factors. In the individual case, different loads of the factorial sets might influence such important clinical characteristics as age at onset, course, and clinical symptomatology. Thusfar, there is no reliable way to discriminate between the A and B sets of factors by means of unanimous clinical indicators. Age at onset is certainly insufficient; an individual manifesting early seizures under the influence of A genes will irretrievably be classified as an A proband, although the later course may well be determined by B genes, in which case the effects would escape detection if only the index case is considered. Moreover, one of the two liabilities may, as a subthreshold character, influence the expression of the above-threshold trait. Finally, lesional factors may interact with these genetic dispositions and lead, for example, to an anticipated expression of a B liability.

At the end of this section, an interesting observation by Seyfried [24] should be mentioned. In inbred strains of mice precipitating audiogenic seizures, two different strains were obtained in backcross experiments. Unlike the original lines, these offspring were susceptible to audiogenic seizures either in the juvenile or in the mature phase. In other words, there were two offspring lines differing as to their age of susceptibility to audiogenic seizures. Obviously, this is due to several threshold factors, each influencing different stages of maturation, and, if present in one individual, sustaining convulsibility over a longer period of time. The segregation of seizure susceptibility, as demonstrated in this experiment, is a convincing analogy to the segregation of A and B factors in the series by Doose and Baier [11].

These considerations are rather hypothetical as long as there are no reliable markers of the different genetic liabilities. In a preliminary conclusion, this study settles some points, but opens many more. It is still impossible to formulate a generally valid concept of the genetics of absence epilepsies. Future concepts will definitely have to consider genetic heterogeneity. A more complete image can be expected from further studies considering the whole variety of primarily generalized seizures, including pure grand mal epilepsies, juvenile myoclonic epilepsy, and febrile convulsions.

Summary

The symptomatological term "absence" does not reflect a nosological entity. For practical reasons, three types of epilepsies in which absences are the principal sign can be differentiated. These are the absence epilepsies of early childhood and of later childhood, and juvenile epilepsy with absences. These disorders are different with respect to symptomatology, therapeutic response, and final outcome. Moreover, they are genetically heterogeneous. Unlike the other types, absences in early childhood are genetically related to seizures of an early onset in the families (including febrile convulsions). Considering all types of epilepsies with absences, the risk in patients' siblings is largely due to "maternal effects." A consistent theory to explain the genetic pathogenesis of epilepsies with absences cannot yet be formulated. However, some of the data are in alignment with predictions obtained under the "multifactorial isocorrelational model."

References

1. Andermann E, Dansky L, Andermann F, Metrakos JD, Metrakos K (1982) EEG in children of epileptic parents: findings and implications. In: Janz D et al. (eds) Epilepsy, pregnancy and the child. Raven Press, New York, pp 457–467
2. Annegers JF, Hauser WA, Elveback LR, Anderson VE, Kurland LT (1976) Seizure disorders in offspring of parents with a history of seizures – a maternal-paternal difference? Epilepsia 17:1–9
3. Bancaud J, Henriksen O, Rubio-Donnadieu F, Seino M, Dreifuss FE, Penry JK (1981) Proposal for revised clinical and electroencephalographic classification of epileptic seizures. Epilepsia 22:489–501
4. Beck-Mannagetta G, Janz D (1982) Febrile convulsions in offspring of epileptic probands. In: Anderson VE, Hauser WA, Penry JK, Sing CF (eds) Genetic basis of the epilepsies. Raven, New York, pp 145–150
5. Beck-Mannagetta G, Janz D (1985) Bedingungen für die Manifestation einer genetischen Anfallsbereitschaft. In: Hallen O, Meyer-Wahl JG, Braun J (eds) Epilepsie 83. Einhorn Presse, Reinbek, pp 32–39
6. Benninger CK, Matthis P, Scheffner D (1982) EEG findings in children of epileptic parents. In: Anderson VE, Hauser WA, Penry JK, Sing CF (eds) Genetic basis of the epilepsies. Raven, New York, pp 95–99
7. Cloninger RC (1986) Personal communication
8. Doose H, Völzke E, Scheffner D (1965) Verlaufsformen kindlicher Epilepsien mit spike wave-Absencen. Arch Psychiat Nervenkr 207:394–415
9. Doose H, Gerken H, Leonhardt R, Völzke E, Völz Ch (1970) Centrencephalic myoclonic-astatic petit mal. Neuropaediatr 2:59–78
10. Doose H, Gerken H, Horstmann T, Völzke E (1973) Genetic factors in spike wave absences. Epilepsia 14:57–75
11. Doose H, Baier WK (1987) Genetic factors in epilepsies with primarily generalized minor seizures. Neuropediatrics 18 (Supplement I):1–64

12. Hauser WA, Chern MM, Anderson VE, Mayersdorf A (1980) Seizure history in families: factors affecting sibling risk for seizures. In: Wada JA, Penry JK (eds) Advances in epileptology: the Xth international symposium. Raven, New York, pp 165–169
13. Janz D (1955) Die klinische Stellung der Pyknolepsie. Dtsch Med Wochenschr 80:1392–1394, 1399–1400
14. Janz D, Beck-Mannagetta G (1982) Epilepsy and neonatal seizures in the offspring of parents with epilepsy. In: Anderson VE, Hauser WA, Penry JK, Sing CF (eds) Genetic basis of the epilepsies. Raven, New York, pp 135–144
15. Janz D, Beck-Mannagetta G, Scheffner D, Scholz G (1982) Epilepsy in children of epileptic parents. In: Janz D, Dam M, Richens A, Bossi L, Helge H, Schmidt D (eds) Epilepsy, pregnancy and the child. Raven, New York, pp 527–534
16. Jung R (1939) Elektroenzephalographische Befunde bei der Epilepsie und ihren Grenzgebieten. Arch Psychiat 109:335–338
17. Lennox WG (1951) The heredity of epilepsy as told by relatives and twins. J Am Med Assoc 146:529–536
18. Lennox WG (1960) Epilepsy and related disorders. Little, Brown, Boston
19. Matthes A, Weber H (1968) Klinische und elektroenzephalographische Familienuntersuchungen bei Pyknolepsien. Dtsch Med Wochenschr 93:429–435
20. Metrakos JD, Metrakos K (1960) Genetics of convulsive disorders. I. Introduction, problems, methods, and base lines. Neurology (Minneap) 10:228–240
21. Metrakos K, Metrakos JD (1961) Genetics of convulsive disorders. II. Genetic and electroencephalographic studies in centrencephalic epilepsy. Neurology (Minneap) 11:464–483
22. Ottman R, Hauser WA, Susser M (1985) Genetic and maternal influences on susceptibility to seizures. Am J Epidemiol 122:923–939
23. Pache HD (1950) Zum Krankheitsbild der kindlichen Pyknolepsie. Verh Dtsch Ges Inn Med, pp 96–98
24. Seyfried TN (1982) Developmental genetics of audiogenic seizure susceptibility in mice. In: Anderson VE, Hauser WA, Penry JK, Sing CF (eds) Genetic basis of the epilepsies. Raven, New York, pp 199–210
25 Tissot SA (1770) Traité de l'epilepsie, faisant le tome troisième du traité des nerfs et de leurs maladies. Paris
26. Tsuboi T (1982) Seizures in children of epileptic parents. In: Akimoto H, Kazamatsuri H, Seino M, Ward A (eds) Advances in epileptology. XIIIth international symposium. Raven, New York, pp 425–428
27. Tsuboi T (1982) Incidence of seizures among offspring of epileptic parents. In: Janz D, Bossi L, Dam M, Helge H, Richens A, Schmidt D (eds) Epilepsy, pregnancy, and the child. Raven, New York, pp 503–507
28. Tsuboi T, Endo S (1977) Incidence of seizures and EEG anomalies among offspring of epileptic patients. Hum Genet 36:173–189

Family Studies on the Genetics of Juvenile Myoclonic Epilepsy (Epilepsy with Impulsive Petit Mal)

D. Janz [1], M. Durner [1], G. Beck-Mannagetta [1], and G. Pantazis [1]

Introduction

The key to success in genetic studies seems to lie in defining simple clinical criteria which appear to be genetically homogeneous. With respect to epilepsy, which is certainly not a nosological entity based on one single criterion, the purpose is therefore to define clinical subtypes which are characterized by as few simple and calculable criteria as possible.

Impulsive petit mal epilepsy (IPM), also known as juvenile myoclonic epilepsy (JME), seems to fulfill such conditions. The epilepsies with absences show a polymorphous pattern of seizures and are very variable as regards age of onset, frequency of seizures, and prognosis. By contrast, JME has a typical clinical leading symptom, namely matutinal jerks. These are irregular, sudden jerks, mainly of both arms and shoulders, experienced shortly after awakening, the patient being conscious. This type of seizure, which we have named impulsive petit mal [12] (a minor epileptic seizure in the form of a sudden jerk – the Latin word is "impulsio"), is the pathognomonic symptom of the subtype of generalized epilepsy named juvenile myoclonic epilepsy [6, 15].

Clinically, and probably genetically, JME is closely related to three further subtypes of generalized epilepsy: childhood absence epilepsy (epilepsy with pyknoleptic absences), juvenile absence epilepsy (epilepsy with nonpyknoleptic absences), and epilepsy with grand mal on awakening. All these subtypes have similar ages of onset: the peak in childhood absences is at the age of 7–8 years, in juvenile absences at 10–14 years, and in JME at 12–18 years (Fig. 1). For grand mal on awakening, the range is much broader: in two-thirds of the cases in one study [14], the epilepsy became manifest between the ages of 9 and 24 years.

The incidence of JME varies according to the age of the patients (Table 1). Bamberger and Matthes [3] found it in only 3.1% of a sample from a children's hospital; Tsuboi and Christian [21], on the other hand, found it in 7.5% of patients in the epilepsy clinic of the Department of Neurology in Heidelberg, while a proportion of nearly 12% was seen in Berlin at a neurological clinic with mainly adult patients [11]. This pattern contrasts with that for the generalized epilepsies of early childhood – that is, the West and Lennox-Gastaut syndromes which were seen by the pediatricians Bamberger and Matthes in 13.4% of all patients with epilepsy, while the incidence in neurological hospitals was only 2.7–3.9% [11, 14,

[1] Neurologische Abteilung, Universitätsklinikum Rudolf Virchow, Freie Universität Berlin, Spandauer Damm 130, D-1000 Berlin 19.

Genetics of the Epilepsies
Beck-Mannagetta et al. (Eds.)

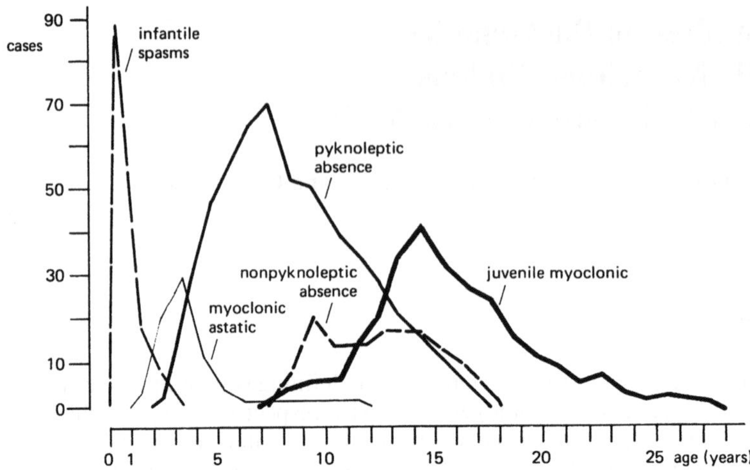

Fig. 1. Subtypes of generalized epilepsy: age of onset. (According to Janz [14], p 149)

Table 1. Subtypes of generalized epilepsy: incidence (%)

	Bamberger and Matthes [3] (n=466)	Janz [14] (n=6 500)	Tsuboi and Christian [21] (n=466)	Wolf and Goosses [23] (n=1 044)
Infantile spasms	13.4	1.8 } 2.9	2.7	3.9
Myoclonic astatic		1.1		
Childhood absence	12.9	7.8 } 10.8	15	9.0 } 16.7
Juvenile absence		3.0		7.7
Juvenile myoclonic	3.1	4.3	7.5	11.6

21]. It is remarkable that the two types of idiopathic absence epilepsy occur with approximately the same frequency, namely 11–17%, in pediatric and neurological departments. Therefore, one can assume that the proportion of JME in a nonselected population of epileptic patients is 7–9%, and thus equal to the proportion of each of the two subtypes of absence epilepsy.

In the subtypes with minor seizures, the EEG patterns showing ictal and interictal bilateral synchronous spike-wave discharges differ only in frequency. This is 3 Hz in childhood absences, somewhat faster and usually combined with double spikes in juvenile absences, and 4–6 Hz and often showing polyspike waves in JME.

With regard to etiology, approximately the same familial proportion of seizures has been reported in all subtypes of generalized epilepsy; however there is no pedigree study with comparable data on incidence and type of seizures and epilepsy in all subgroups. The question therefore remains unanswered as to whether the quartet of idiopathic generalized epilepsies briefly described above represents one genetic entity or whether each subtype is a specific genetic entity on its own.

Clinical Data

We report on 181 patients (77 male and 104 female) with the common symptom of matutinal jerks; 13 (7.2%) had only jerks, the others had generalized tonic-clonic seizures (TCS) in addition, occurring predominantly after awakening. The disease almost always started with jerks (42%) or with jerks and TCS at the same time (35%), and only in 23% with major seizures. Fifty-one patients (28.2%) had absences as well. (In then cases pyknoleptic, i.e. daily, absences occurred; in 39 cases nonpyknoleptic absences. In two cases we do not know the frequency of the absences.)

The age of onset was between 12 and 19 years in 80% of cases. Jerks occurred for the first time at an average age of 15.3; major seizures at an average age of 16.6 years.

In JME, the EEG most frequently showed a polyspike-wave (PSW) pattern (Table 2). Together with bispike-wave discharges, PSWs occur in our study, as in

Table 2. EEG in JME: spike-wave (SW) activity

Paroxysmal activity	Our study (181 cases)		Tsuboi [22] (381 cases)		Delgado-Escueta and Enrile-Bacsal [6] (43 cases)		Simonsen et al. [19] (35 cases)		Asconapé and Penry [2] (12 cases)	
	n	%	*n*	%	*n*	%	*n*	%	*n*	%
PSW	89	49.2	104	27.3						
		59.7		37.3			31	88.6	7	58.3
BSW	19	10.5	41	11.0						
PSW+BSW+SW4–6 Hz	124	68.5			43	100.0				
SW except PSW+BSW	32	17.7	122	32.0						
Total SW	140	77.4	267	70.1	43	100.0				

PSW, polyspike wave; BSW, bispike wave; SW, spike wave.

Table 3. EEG in different types of epilepsy: spike-wave (SW) activity. (From [21])

Paroxysmal activity	Type of seizures						Control (466 cases)
	Juvenile myoclonic (381 cases) %	Awakening grand mal (147 cases) %	Ab-sences (70 cases) %	Sleep grand mal (89 cases) %	Psycho-motor (119 cases) %	Neo-cortical (40 cases) %	%
PSW+BSW	37.3	16.3	18.6	0	1.7	2.5	7.1
3.5–5/s SW	21.5	9.5	11.4	1.1	0.8	2.5	5.4
3/s SW	11.0	12.9	18.6	0	1.7	2.5	5.1
Other SW	15.2	13.6	15.7	0	3.4	2.5	4.5
Total SW	70.1	33.3	37.1	1.1	7.6	7.5	16.3

PSW, polyspike wave; BSW, bispike wave.

Asconapé and Penry's [2] in 58% of cases; in the study by Simonsen et al. [19] the incidence was as high as 88.6%. As to the frequency of spike-wave discharges, fast spike waves were registered by Tsuboi and Christian [21] in 58.8% of cases, in the present study in 68.5%, and by Delgado-Escueta and Enrile-Bacsal [6] in 100%. The only comparison of corresponding data in other kinds of epilepsy was presented in 1976 by Tsuboi and Christian [21] (Table 3). Their study shows that all spike-wave patterns faster than 3 Hz also occur in other idiopathic generalized epilepsies, but significantly less frequently. This seems to relativize the specificity of the PSW pattern to the subtype JME. However, as long as the study design does not allow those probands with additional jerks to be excluded from the probands with the two other types of idiopathic generalized epilepsy in which Tsuboi and Christian were able to register fast SW patterns, the assumption can be held that at least the PSW pattern is specific for JME.

Another EEG criterion which seems to be relatively specific to JME is "photosensitivity", or the precipitation of a bilateral synchronous SW pattern by flickering light. This genetically determined bioelectrical reaction has been found significantly more frequently in JME than in the other subtypes of idiopathic generalized epilepsy [11, 23] (Table 4). It should be noted that this difference is due to the preponderance of female patients. The preponderance of females among patients showing photosensitivity has already been shown by Doose et al. [8], but in JME it is seen only among patients without absences.

Clinical Genetics

The proportion of patients with JME having close or distant relatives with seizures was between 25% and 30% in the studies with a larger number of cases (Table 5). In all studies, the majority of patients with affected relatives was female. In 466 nonselected patients with epilepsy of all kinds, Tsuboi and Christian [20] found relatives with seizures in only 9.9%. It can therefore be taken for granted that family predisposition in JME is significantly higher than in epilepsy in general. However, there seems to be no significant difference between the vari-

Table 4. Photosensitivity in different types of generalized epilepsy (according to Wolf and Goosses [11])

Epilepsy	Male		Female		Total	
	n	%	*n*	%	*n*	%
Pyknoleptic absence	41	19.5	53	17	94	18
Nonpyknoleptic absences	41	5	39	10	80	7.5
Awakening TCS	127	9	143	17	270	13
Juvenile myoclonic	61	20	60	42	121	30.5

TCS, tonic-clonic seizures.

Table 5. Proportion of JME patients with relatives who had seizures

	Total *n* of cases	*n*	%
1957 Janz and Christian [13]	47	8	17
1958 Castells and Mendilaharsu [5]	70	26	37
1960 Aigner and Mulder [1]			13
1969 Janz [14]	280	70	25
1973 Tsuboi and Christian [20]	319	87	27
1984 Delgado-Escueta and Enrile-Bacsal [6]	43	17	39
1984 Asconapé and Penry [2]	12	6	50
1985 Gonzalez and Astiazaran	20	14	70
1988 Our study	118	38	32

Table 6. Different types of epilepsy: proportion of patients with relatives who had seizures

	n	%
Generalized epilepsies		
Doose (1964); Propulsive petit mal	71	25
Kruse (1968); Myoclonic astatic petit mal	80	29
Doose et al. (1985); Myoclonic-astatic epilepsy of early childhood	100	37
Matthes & Weber (1968); Pyknoleptic absences	129	32
Doose et al. (1973); 3/sec SW absences	239	30
Symptomatic and focal epilepsies		
Evans (1962); Postraumatic epilepsy	80	7.5
Lund (1952); Tumor epilepsy	966	6
Janz (1969); Psychomotor seizures	1990	6.5
Gibbs & Gibbs (1952); Neocortical seizures	978	6

ous subtypes of generalized and idiopathic epilepsy, only between generalized epilepsies on the one hand and focal and symptomatic epilepsies on the other (Table 6). The figures given provide only very rough and superficial information: febrile and nonfebrile seizures are not separated, numbers and sex of the patients and their relatives are not known, and the degree of relationship is not indicated.

In our study, the number of first-degree relatives (parents, siblings, and children) with epileptic seizures represents a prevalence of 5.5% (Table 7); in Tsuboi and Christian's study 4.1% (5% after age correction; Table 8). In our study, in contrast to Tsuboi and Christian's, female relatives are not significantly more affected, but in both studies the proportion of epileptic relatives of female patients is higher than that of male patients. The fact attracting most attention is that in both studies epilepsy is less prevalent among male relatives of male patients.

It is remarkable that febrile convulsions occur in families of patients with JME in only 1.7% of the cases: less than in the general population and less than in families of patients with absence epilepsy. This relatively rare occurrence is perhaps a further genetically determined differentiation criterion in relation to other subtypes of epilepsy and even to generalized epilepsy. Febrile seizures, too, seem to appear less often in the case histories of patients with JME than in those

Table 7. Incidence of febrile and nonfebrile seizures among first-degree relatives

Probands	Male (51 cases)			Female (67 cases)			Total (118 cases)		
	N	*n*	%	*N*	*n*	%	*N*	*n*	%
Nonfebrile seizures									
Male relatives	3	319	2.2	12	163	7.4	15	302	5.0
Female relatives	7	115	6.1	11	183	6.0	18	298	6.0
Total 1° relatives	10	254	3.9	23	346	6.7	33	600	5.5
Febrile seizures									
Total 1° relatives	6	254	2.3	4	346	1.2	10	600	1.7

Table 8. Incidence of epilepsy among first-degree relatives. (From [20])

Probands	Male (161 cases)			Female (158 cases)			Total (319 cases)		
	N	*n*	%	*N*	*n*	%	*N*	*n*	%
Male relatives	5	411	1.2	19	429	4.4	24	840	2.9
Female relatives	11	376	2.9	31	402	7.7	42	778	5.4
Total 1° relatives	16	787	2.0	50	831	6.0	66	1618	4.1

of patients with other types of epilepsy, in particular absence epilepsy. Among 65 cases of epilepsy developed after febrile convulsions, we found only one patient with JME, in contrast to 28 patients with absence epilepsy (13 with pyknoleptic and 15 with non-pyknoleptic absences) [4].

As regards the risks for different generations: according to Tsuboi and Christian [20], parents of patients with JME are less frequently affected (3.3%) than siblings (4.4%), and these again less frequently than offspring (5.1%; Table 9). We found approximately the same relationship (Table 10). Among parents, 3.4% were affected with epilepsy, but with no predominance of mothers. The proportion of epilepsy among siblings is a bit more in our study (5.0%) to that in Tsuboi and Christian's. It is similar with regard to the difference between the siblings of male and female patients: both studies show that siblings of female patients run a two- to threefold risk of developing epilepsy compared to siblings of male patients. In contrast to Tsuboi and Christian, we found brothers of female patients more often affected than sisters. This is similar to the findings in parents, where fathers of female patients are more often affected. We can confirm our predecessors' results concerning offspring: epilepsy is to be found in 6.6% of offspring. The risk for daughters is higher than that for sons: according to our study, the incidence in female offspring is almost threefold. Tsuboi and Christian [20] observed a fivefold incidence. We could not confirm that there is a higher risk of recurrence in children of affected mothers than in children of male patients. Daughters of fathers with JME seem to run the highest risk in our study. The figures do not show, however, the real risk of recurrence: most of the children were of an age at which epilepsy has not yet become manifest. These numbers can be corrected by assuming that epilepsy has not yet become apparent in two-thirds of the cases

Table 9. Incidence of epilepsy among parents, siblings and offspring of patients with JME. (From [20])

Probands	Male (161 cases)			Female (158 cases)			Total (319 cases)		
	n	*N*	%	*n*	*N*	%	*n*	*N*	%
Father	2	161	1.2	4	158	2.5	6	319	1.9
Mother	6	161	3.7	9	158	5.7	15	319	4.7
Parents	8	322	2.5	13	316	4.1	21	638	3.3
Brother	3	167	1.8	12	191	6.3	15	358	4.2
Sister	3	165	1.8	13	182	7.1	16	347	4.6
Siblings	6	332	1.8	25	373	6.7	31	705	4.4
Son	0	83	0.0	3	80	3.8	3	163	1.8
Daughter	2	50	4.0	9	62	14.5	11	112	9.8
Offspring	2	133	1.5	12	142	8.5	14	275	5.1

Table 10. Incidence of nonfebrile seizures among parents, siblings and offspring of patients with JME

Probands	Male (51 cases)			Female (67 cases)			Total (118 cases)		
	N	*n*	%	*N*	*n*	%	*N*	*n*	%
Father	0	51	0	4	67	6.0	4	118	3.4
Mother	2	51	3.9	2	67	3.0	4	118	3.4
Parents	2	102	2.0	6	134	4.5	8	236	3.4
Brother	2	65	3.1	7	67	10.4	9	132	6.8
Sister	3	55	5.4	7	86	8.1	10	141	7.1
Siblings	5	120	4.2	14	153	9.2	19	273	7.0
Son	1	23	4.3	1	29	3.5	2	52	3.8
Daughter	2	9	22.2	2	30	6.7	4	39	10.3
Children	3	31	9.7	3	59	5.1	6	91	6.6

up to the age of ten and in one-third up to the age of 20. After this correction, Tsuboi and Christian [20] expect that one-sixth of all children and one-fourth of all daughters will be affected by epilepsy.

Evidence concerning genetic independence of JME or its genetic relationship with other subtypes of generalized epilepsy can be deduced from the proportions of the different types of epilepsy among the affected relatives of patients with JME (Table 11). Tsuboi and Christian [20] found JME in 15% of the near and distant relatives with epilepsy. This rate is approximately twice as high as in a nonselected epilepsy population (33/466 = 7.1%). The incidence of epilepsies with pyknoleptic (childhood) and nonpyknoleptic (juvenile) absences (14.6%) correlated well with the expectation (70/466 = 15.0%). In Delgado-Escueta and Enrile-Bacsal's series [6] JME also appeared in first-degree relatives as often as the two kinds of absence epilepsy. In our study, JME represents one-third and absences one-fourth of all epilepsies in first-degree relatives. As mentioned above the frequency of each of the three subtypes – childhood absence epilepsy, juvenile ab-

Table 11. Types of seizures in first degree relatives of 100 patients with JME

Type of seizure	Our study		Tsuboi and Christian [20]		Delgado-Escueta and Enrile-Bascal [6]
	n	%	*n*	%	*n*
IPM	10	30	17	15	5
Absences	9	26	7	15	5
Myoclonic-astatic			1	1	
TCS	14	41	99	85	11
Complex focal	1	3	1	1	

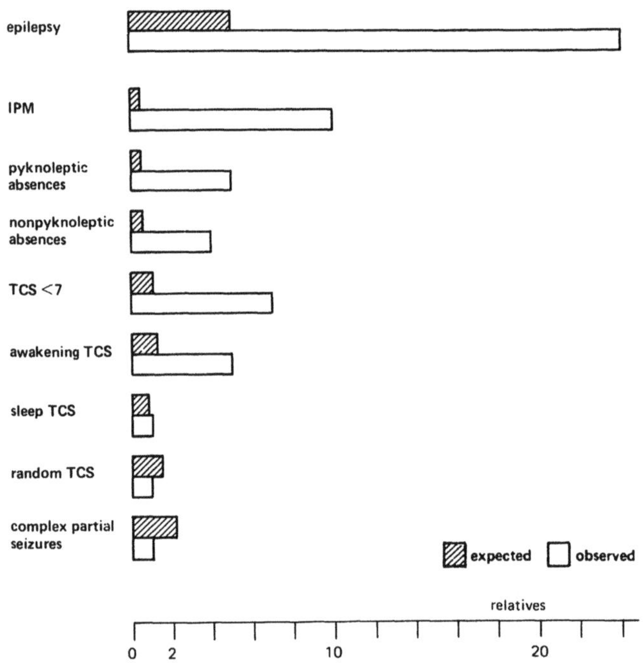

Fig. 2. Types of seizures ($n=34$) in first-degree relatives ($n=501$) of 100 patients with JME. In cases with combinations of seizures, each type is registered separately. *TCS*, tonic-clonic seizure

sence epilepsy, and JME – is around 8% of all epilepsies. JME thus occurs in first-degree relatives four times more frequently than expected and absences twice as frequently.

JME occurs in the general population at the rate of about 0.1%. It is found in first-degree relatives of our patients twenty times more frequently, and absences ten times more frequently (Fig. 2). When awakening TCSs are excluded, other types of generalized epilepsy, especially focal epilepsies, are of no importance.

On the basis of these findings, a close genetic relationship between the three subtypes of idiopathic generalized epilepsy seems to be certain. The greater prevalence of JME suggests a certain genetic specificity of JME.

It will be the aim of future studies to find out which clinical and electroencephalographical characteristics are specific to JME and which are shared with the other subtypes of idiopathic generalized epilepsy.

Summary

Of all forms of idiopathic epilepsy, juvenile myoclonic epilepsy (JME), also called impulsive petit mal epilepsy (IPM), seems to show the greatest clinical and electroencephalographical homogeneity. Nevertheless, a close relationship exists between JME and both epilepsies with childhood and juvenile absences.

The proportion of fast spike waves and polyspike waves in the EEG of JME patients is higher than in other subtypes. Photosensitivity is significantly more frequent, particularly in female probands. Genetic predisposition does not exceed that of other forms of epilepsy with an age-dependent onset of minor seizures. First-degree relatives of female patients are more affected by nonfebrile seizures than relatives of males. The sex ratio of affected relatives is balanced. The lowest rate of affected family members is observed in male relatives of male patients with JME. Parents are less often affected than siblings, and these again less frequently than offspring. There is no difference in the sex distribution of affected parents and siblings of male patients, while in the case of female patients we have found (in contrast to findings reported in the literature) that males predominate among relatives with seizures. Children of fathers with JME are more frequently affected by nonfebrile seizures than children of mothers with JME. Nonfebrile seizures are observed particulary often in daughters of fathers with JME. As regards seizure type, febrile convulsions occur less often than expected in close relatives and in patients with JME themselves. In comparison to what would be expected in the general population, the frequency of JME in first-degree relatives is increased twentyfold and that of absences, tenfold. Among all the subtypes of epilepsy observed in close relatives, JME is found three times and absences one-and-a-half times more often than in a population of unselected patients with epilepsy. There seems to be a relatively specific transmission of JME within families.

Acknowledgement. This study was supported by the Deutsche Forschungsgemeinschaft.

References

1. Aigner BR, Mulder DW (1960) Myoclonus. Clinical significance and an approach to classification. Arch Neurol (Chicago) 2:600–615
2. Asconapé J, Penry K (1984) Some clinical and EEG aspects of benign juvenile myoclonic epilepsy. Epilepsia 25:108–114
3. Bamberger P, Matthes A (1959) Anfälle im Kindesalter. Karger, Basel
4. Beck-Mannagetta G, Hensen J, Janz D (1987) Seizure type in epileptic patients with a history of febrile convulsions. In: Wolf P, Janz D, Dreifuss F, Dam M (eds) Advances in epileptology. 16th Epilepsy international symposium. Raven, New York

5. Castells C, Mendilaharsu C (1958) La epilepsia mioclónica bilateral y consciente. Acta Neurol Latinoamer 4:23–48
6. Delgado-Escueta AV, Enrile-Bacsal FE (1984) Juvenile myoclonic epilepsy of Janz. Neurology 34:285–294
7. Doose H (1964) Zur Nosologie der Blitz-Nick-Salaamkrämpfe. Arch Psychiat Nervenkr 206:28-48
8. Doose H, Gerken H, Hien-Völpel KF, Völzke E (1969) Genetics of photosensitive epilepsy. Neuropädiatrie 1:56–73
9. Doose H (1985) Myoclonic astatic epilepsy of early childhood. In: Roger J, Dravet C, Bureau M, Dreifuss FE, Wolf P (eds) Epileptic syndromes in infancy, childhood and adolescence. Libbey, London
10. Gibbs FA, Gibbs EL (1952) Atlas of electroencephalography. Addison Wesley, Cambridge, Mass
11. Goosses R (1984) Die Beziehung der Fotosensibilität zu verschiedenen epileptischen Syndromen. Dissertation, Berlin
12. Janz D (1955) Die Petit mal-Epilepsien. Thesis, Heidelberg
13. Janz D, Christian W (1957) Impulsiv-Petit mal. Dtsch Z Nervenheilk 176:346–386
14. Janz D (1969) Die Epilepsien. Spezielle Pathologie und Therapie. Thieme, Stuttgart
15. Janz D (1985) Epilepsy with impulsive petit mal (juvenile myoclonic epilepsy). Acta Neurol Scand 72:449–459
16. Kruse R (1968) Das myoklonisch-astatische Petit mal. Springer, Berlin Heidelberg New York
17. Lund M (1952) Epilepsy in association with intracranial tumor. Acta Psychiat Scand [Suppl] 18
18. Matthes A, Weber H (1968) Klinische und elektroencephalographische Familienuntersuchungen bei Pyknolepsien. Dtsch Med Wochenschr 93:429–435
19. Simonsen N, Møllgaard V, Lund M (1976) A controlled clinical and electroencephalographic study of myoclonic epilepsy (Impulsiv-Petit mal). In: Janz D (ed) Epileptology. Thieme, Stuttgart, pp 41–48
20. Tsuboi T, Christian W (1973) On the genetics of the primary generalized epilepsy with sporadic myoclonias of impulsive petit mal type. Humangenetik 19:155–182
21. Tsuboi T, Christian W (1976) A clinical, electroencephalographic and statistical study of 466 patients. (Neurology series) Springer, Berlin Heidelberg New York
22. Tsuboi T (1977) Primary generalized epilepsy with sporadic myoclonias of myoclonic petit mal type. A clinical, electroencephalographic, statistical and genetic study of 399 probands. Thieme, Stuttgart
23. Wolf P, Goosses R (1986) Relation of photosensitivity to epileptic syndromes. J Neurol Neurosurg Psychiat 49:1386–1391

Segregation Analysis of Juvenile Myoclonic Epilepsy

D. A. Greenberg [1], A. V. Delgado-Escueta [2], H. H. Maldonado [3], and H. Widelitz [1]

We have been collecting data, including EEG information, on juvenile myoclonic epilepsy (JME) families for the past several years, and this report will discuss the results of our analyses of this family data.

At least since the work of Tsuboi and Christian [13], it has been clear that there is a genetic component to the inheritance of juvenile myoclonic epilepsy or the syndrome of Janz. Despite the fact that JME may comprise between 4% and 10% of all epilepsy [3, 6, 11], the relatively low prevalence has made it difficult to study. Even more of a problem has been the fact that, until the last few years, it was not recognized as a distinct clinical entity even by epileptologists.

The focus of this report is the segregation analysis of the JME family data, which includes EEG information on family members as well as whether family members are affected with clinical epilepsy or not. The EEG findings are important because they provide us with a subclinical marker for what we believe to be at least part of the disease genotype.

Segregation Analysis

To begin with, let us define segregation analysis.[4] Segregation analysis tests whether the family data of a disease or trait are consistent with a specific mode of inheritance. In segregation analysis we *assume* a certain genetic model for some disease or trait, and then we test whether the data that we have gathered *reject* that assumed model.

Criteria used for Definings JME for the study

Table 1 shows the criteria we used in deciding to whether include a person in the study. While some epileptologists might consider these criteria overly restrictive,

[1] Southwest Regional VA Epilepsy Center, Neurology Service, Wadsworth VA Medical Center, Los Angeles. Current address: Department of Psychiatry, Mt. Sinai Medical Center, 1 Gustave Levy Place, New York, NY 10029, USA.

[2] Reed Neurological Research Center, UCLA School of Medicine, 710 Westwood Plaza, Los Angeles, CA 90024, USA.

[3] Southwest Regional VA Epilepsy Center, Neurology Service, Wadsworth VA Medical Center, Los Angeles, CA 90073, USA.

[4] Segregation analysis should not be confused with a risk analysis. Simple risk analysis does not attempt to test how the disease is inherited but calculates, based on family history information, what the risk is for any relative to develop epilepsy.

Genetics of the Epilepsies
Beck-Mannagetta et al. (Eds.)

Table 1. Definition of JME

Myoclonic jerks occurring most often shortly after awakening
Age of onset between 10 and 25 years – most often about 15
Associated generalized seizures (tonic-clonic and, sometimes, juvenile absences)
No history of onset after head trauma, encephalitis, etc.
No family history of degenerative myoclonus epilepsy
No mental retardation
No evidence of degenerative disease

such a definition of JME is necessary in order to try and eliminate other, apparently similar syndromes from the data. One of the greatest problems in genetic analysis is that of heterogeneity – that is, where there are two or more diseases of differing etiologies that appear to be the same. A familiar example of this is insulin-dependent diabetes vs. noninsulin dependent diabetes. Here are two conditions that have compelling similarities yet also have distinct differences. It has been only in the last 20 years that it was conclusively demonstrated, through genetic analysis, that there are at least three different conditions that are called diabetes. Any genetic analyses that were done on the undifferentiated condition of "diabetes" were doomed to failure because of this heterogeneity. We do not claim that we have eliminated all possibility of heterogeneity in our data by using these criteria for inclusion in the study, but that possibility is reduced.

Epilepsy Data

We studied 28 families in our segregation analysis. Of these, 22 had complete or partial EEG information.

There was one family multiplex for JME, two families multiplex for JME and another form of epilepsy, and two with a parent with epilepsy or a history of seizures. We counted someone with a history of seizures as affected if they had more than one unexplained seizure and/or were taking antiepileptic drugs. In fact, there was no instance of ambiguity of classification in the current data set.

Abnormal EEGs

Seven sibs of probands who were not clinically affected (out of 41 tested) had abnormal EEGs. Two parents of probands (out of 38 tested) had abnormal EEGs.

The EEG abnormalities found were mostly a diffuse rhythmic slowing of 3–6 Hz. Two of the sibs had the 4–6 Hz multispike and wave (MS&W) trait also seen interictally in JME patients. (We will discuss the frequency of these traits in the general population below.)

Analyses

Because of the variety of our data, we examined the data in two ways. First, we classified those relatives as affected who had overt epilepsy and we classified the people with abnormal EEGs as unaffected. Second, we also classified the abnormal EEGs as affected.

We tested several models of inheritance, viz. the single locus recessive model and several two-locus models. Under the recessive model, an affected person must have a disease allele on each chromosome in order to be affected with the disease. The two-locus models make the assumption that there are two gene loci involved in the inheritance of the disease and that there are two alleles at each locus. Furthermore, the inheritance at each locus is assumed to be either dominant or recessive.

We considered the two-locus models when trying to account for so-called reduced penetrance. Reduced penetrance generally means that we find that the segregation ratio is less than the expected 0.25 for recessive and/or 0.5 for dominant inheritance. The finding that the segregation ratio does not meet our expectations with regard to the single-locus mendelian models means that we must consider other models. The two-locus models are the next-simplest models after the single locus dominant and recessive models. We will discuss the two-locus models below.

A Crude Approximation

Before we proceed to the findings of the formal segregation analysis, let us do a simple calculation which gives us an approximation of the segregation ratio. The segregation ratio is the proportion of sibs affected from *all at-risk matings* – including those that produced no affected offspring. Because families with zero affected people do not seek medical help for epilepsy, we need to correct for these "missing" data. This correction is called ascertainment bias correction. Weinberg [14] described a simple method for ascertainment correction when there was only one proband per family. In order to calculate this estimate of the segregation ratio, one takes the number of affected sibs minus the number of probands and divides by the total number of sibs minus the probands. This calculation takes into account neither gene frequency considerations nor parental mating type, but gives a good first approximation of the segregation ratio if the mode of ascertainment is single [8].

When we do this calculation using our data, not including the EEG data, the segregation ration (SR) is:

$$SR = \frac{31-28}{107-28} = 0.04$$

and if we include the EEG data:

$$SR = \frac{32-22}{77-22} = 0.18 .$$

Segregation ratios of 0.04 and 0.18 both fall short of the expected 0.25 for simple recessive inheritance. But can one *statistically* reject the simple recessive model? In order to answer this question, we proceed with a formal segregation analysis [9]. This will also allow us to take into account parental affectedness status as well as the influence of gene frequency assumptions.

Results Assuming Single-Locus Recessive

We tested a range of gene frequencies from 0.01 to 0.2. Table 2 shows the segregation ratio for the data taking the abnormal EEGs as *not affected.* The segregation ratio we calculate is not terribly different from what we got from our simple calculation and also not very dependent on the assumed gene frequency. Here, the chi-square was 20 with one degree of freedom ($p < 0.0001$), which is a clear rejection of the fully penetrant recessive when we classify the abnormal EEGs as unaffected.

If we now classify the abnormal EEGs as affected, we get a segregation ratio of between 0.15 and 0.14 (Table 3). Here, the chi-square was also significant ($p < 0.01$), which also rejects the fully penetrant recessive.

We can conclude, based on the current data, that the fully penetrant recessive can be rejected even if we classify the abnormal EEGs as affected.

What would explain the reduced penetrance? One obvious answer involves environmental factors. It is possible that this is a factor in the epilepsy itself, although we have tried to eliminate environment as a component by not including people with a history of head trauma associated with the onset of seizures. But the silent EEG abnormalities are more difficult to explain environmentally. There is always the possibility of simply random factors – that is, the abnormalities do not show up sometimes even though the genetic substrate is there. This hypothesis can only be proved by elimination of all other possibilities. A hypothesis more amenable to testing is one involving other genetic factors.

We went on to test whether two genes could be interacting to produce either the epilepsy alone of the epilepsy plus EEG traits.

Two-Locus Models

The two-locus models that we looked at were simple ones. We assume that there are two genetic loci and that there are two alleles at each locus, one normal allele and one trait (or disease) allele. The mode of inheritance at each locus is assumed to be either dominant or recessive. This leads to three different two-locus models: the double recessive, the double dominant, and one dominant and one recessive

Table 2. Results of segregation analysis classifying the abnormal EEGs as *unaffected*

Assumed gene frequency	0.01 → 0.2
Resulting segregation ratio	0.04 → 0.03

$\chi^2 = 20$ (1 degree of freedom).

Table 3. Results of segregation analysis classifying the abnormal EEGs as *affected*

Assumed gene frequency	0.01 → 0.2
Resulting segregation ratio	0.15 → 0.14

$\chi^2 = 5$ (1 degree of freedom).

Table 4. Lowest possible segregation ratio for the three two-locus models

Model	Lowest segregation ratio possible
Recessive–recessive	0.0625
Dominant–dominant	0.25
Dominant–recessive	0.125

locus. These models have certain mathematical limits associated with them. The lowest possible segregation ratios that each can have is shown in Table 4. As you can see, the data on the epilepsy alone, that is not counting the abnormal EEGs as affected – which gave a segregation ratio of about 0.04 with both the simple calculation and the formal segregation analysis – is lower than the lowest possible prediction of all three models. Therefore, the two-locus models will not explain the data if the data include only the family members with epilepsy.

For the EEG plus epilepsy data, the double dominant is eliminated because we observe a segregation ratio of between 0.14 and 0.18, which is lower than the lowest possible segregation ratio for the double dominant. But the double recessive and the dominant recessive are not eliminated on the basis of the lowest possible segregation ratio.

We have developed graphs [7] that test two-locus inheritance easily. We need two pieces of information in order to do this test. One is the segregation ratio, which we have, and the other is the population prevalence for the trait under discussion. Details of how these graphs were derived can be found in [7]. Briefly, each point on the population prevalence graph was obtained by using the gene frequencies at the two loci (as indicated on the axes, see figures) to calculate the population prevalence. Similarly, the segregation ratio is a function of the two-gene frequencies at each locus and is shown on the segregation ratio graph. What we test is whether the prevalence data and the segregation ratio data are compatible with each other, that is, do the gene frequencies that lead to the observed population prevalence lead to the observed segregation ratio? If we mark on the graphs what areas are delimited by the observed population prevalence and segregation ratio (the shaded areas on the prevalence and segregation ratio graphs, Fig. 1 and 2), then we have defined a set of gene frequency combinations that is consistent with the observed values of those parameters. We can then overlay the population prevalence and segregation ratio graphs to see whether the compatible gene frequencies match (the overlap graphs in Fig. 1 and 2). If they do not overlap, then the gene frequencies leading to the observed population prevalence do not lead to the observed segregation ratio and the model being tested is rejected. If they do overlap then the model is not rejected.

As discussed above, the range for the segregation ratio that we observe is between 0.13 and 0.18, depending on the gene frequency. The population prevalence is somewhat problematic because population prevalence figures on EEG abnormalities are difficult to interpret. However, almost all studies agree on a figure of about 0.05 for the prevalence of *all* nonspecific, paroxysmal EEG abnormali-

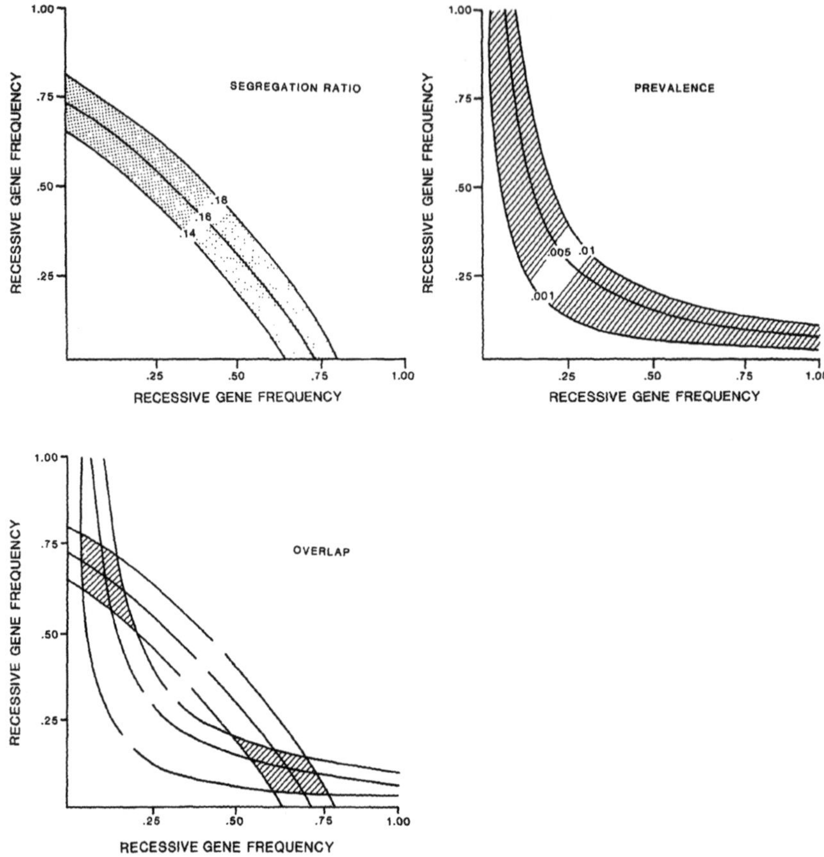

Fig. 1. Recessive–recessive model

ties in the general population [2, 10, 12, 13]. The paroxysmal EEG abnormalities in these reports usually include focal abnormalites, which we did not consider in our study. The age distribution in the studies also varied, but generally included a younger population than was in our population of family members (in our families, the youngest sib we studied was 20 years old). We also know from the work of Doose et al. [5] that the frequency of the kind of EEG abnormality that we see in these families, a 3–6 Hz high amplitude theta slowing, is seen in less than 1% of the population over the age of 18. Tsuboi and Christian [13], who also studied a control population, found a maximum of 6% EEG abnormalities, including many different kinds of EEG abnormalities. These factors make a value of 0.05 for the population prevalence somewhat high. Since we are considering the EEG trait as being a form of affected, and it is the most common manifestation of the

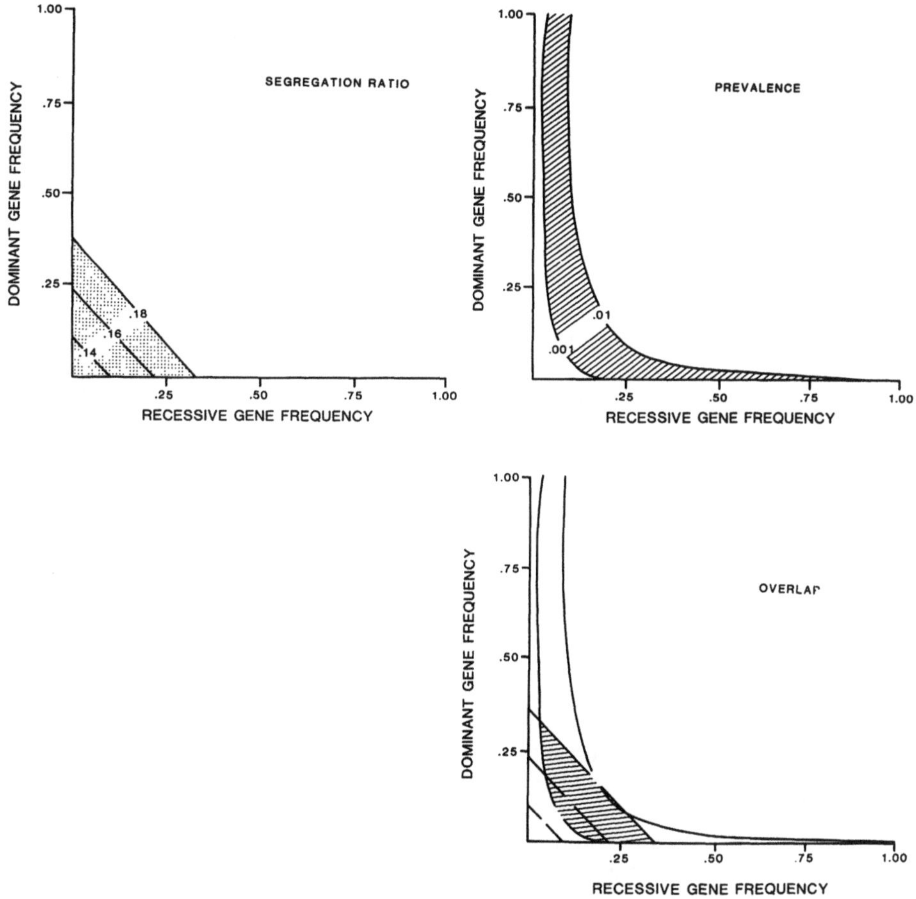

Fig. 2. Dominant–recessive model

proposed genes, we used a population prevalence figure of 0.01, or 1 in 100, as the upper limit of the population prevalence of the trait. Remember that this is the frequency of the abnormal EEG trait plus epilepsy.

Figure 1 shows the graph for the population prevalence for the double recessive model. On the population prevalence graph, the shaded area shows which population prevalences lie between the observed limits. The segregation ratio graph is shown in a similar manner. If we overlay the two graphs (overlap graph) we see that there is some overlap, but only at the periphery of the graphs. From our experience, this does not especially support a two-locus, double-recessive model. The fact that one of the gene frequencies approaches 1.0 leads one to distrust the conclusion that one gene frequency is simply very high and the other very low. But, it must be said that this is a heuristic argument and not a statistical one.

There has been limited experience with the two-locus methods and we are working towards hardening this heuristic notion.

Now let us look at the model where there is one recessive locus and one dominant locus (Fig. 2). Here we see the overlap is central and almost exactly coincides for the limits on both graphs. I must emphasize this does not prove that a two-locus dominant-recessive model is the answer. It only explains all the data we currently have and gives us a proposed model to try and disprove.

Discussion

If we may be allowed to speculate for a moment, a two-locis dominant-recessive model is a most appealing one for several reasons. First, it allows us to explain findings from a variety of epilepsies and EEG studies. Second, it is a completely genetic model while retaining a variety of possible phenotypes. If we imagine two loci with several possible disease alleles at each locus, combinations of theses alleles could lead to different forms of generalized epilepsy or abnormal EEGs. (In the current analysis, we combined all possible disease-causing or trait alleles into one.) If that were the case, we could, with a single genetic system, account for the occurrence of different forms of epilepsy and abnormal EEGs in the same family. Since a two-locus model is entirely genetic, one would predict that the identical twin concordance rate would be 1.0. While the results of studies of twins with epilepsy are varied, the concordance rates reported have been high [1], and those studies have usually not been as selective in criteria as we have tried to be for the JME study.

To summarize the conclusions of this study: If we look just at people in the families who have epilepsy, all the models we looked at can be rejected. When we include the EEG information, the single-locus recessive can still be rejected. The two-locus double-recessive model, while not statistically rejectable, does not appear as favorable as the two-locus dominant-recessive.

I must emphasize that most of the information we have been using, in terms of family data, comes from the EEG information. Whatever the mode of inheritance, other factors, perhaps other genes or the environment, contribute to the manifestation of the epilepsy itself.

Acknowledgements. This work was supported in part by Grants NS21908 and AM31775 from the National Institutes of Health and by the Veterans Admimistration.

References

1. Anderson VE, Wilcox K, Rich SS, Leppik LE (1987) Twin studies in epilepsy (this volume)
2. Christiani K (1979) Klinisch-elektroenzephalographische Untersuchungen bei Kindern von Epileptikern. Fortschr Neurol Psychiat 47:221–263
3. Delgado-Escueta AV, Enrile-Bascal F (1984) Juvenile myoclonic epilepsy of Janz. Neurology 34:285–294
4. Delgado-Escueta AV, White R, Greenberg DA, Treiman LJ (1986) Looking for epilepsy genes. In: Delgado-Escueta AV, Ward AA, Woodbury DM, Porter RJ (eds) Advances in neurology. Raven, New York, pp 77–95

5. Doose H, Gerken H, Völzke E (1972) On the genetics of EEG-anomalies in childhood. I. Abnormal theta rhythms. Neuropaediatrie 3:386–401
6. Escueta AV, Greenberg DA (1984) The search for epilepsies ideal for clinical and molecular genetic studies. Ann Neurol 16 (Suppl):S1–S11
7. Greenberg DA (1981) A simple method for testing two-locus models of inheritance. Am J Hum Genet 33:519–530
8. Greenberg DA (1984) Simulation studies of segregation analysis: application to two-locus inheritance. Am J Hum Genet 36:167–176
9. Greenberg DA, Lange K (1982) A maximum likelihood test of the two-locus model for coeliac disease. Am J Med Genet 12:75–82
10. Handbook of Electroencephalography and Clinical Neurophysiology (1976) Vol 6, "The Normal EEG Throughout Life." Chatrian GE, Lairy GC (eds), pp 114–118
11. Janz D, Durner M, Beck-Mannagetta, Behl I, Scholz G, Pantazis G (1987) Family studies in juvenile myoclonic epilepsy (this volume)
12. Oberholz H, Kugler J, Jessberger W (1975) EEG criteria for flying fitness applied by the German Air Force Institute of Aviation Medicine. Aviat Space Environ Med 46:194–198
13. Tsuboi T, Christian W (1973) On the genetics of the primary generalized epilepsy with sporadic myoclonias of impulsive petit mal type: a clinical and electroencephalographic study of 399 probands. Humangenetik 19:155–182
14. Weinberg W (1912) Methoden and Fehlerquellen der Untersuchung auf Mendelsche Zahlen beim Menschen. Arch Rassenbiol 9:165–174

Is Juvenile Myoclonic Epilepsy Polygenic?

S. E. Hodge [1], D. A. Greenberg [2], M. Durner [3],
A. V. Delgado-Escueta [4], and D. Janz [3]

It has been suggested [3, 6] that juvenile myoclonic epilepsy (JME) may follow a polygenic threshold pattern of inheritance – specifically, with a differential sex effect, in that females are more often affected than males. However, as described below, we have examined 78 families with JME from Berlin and 27 from Los Angeles and have found no evidence to support the polygenic hypothesis for pure JME, either with or without differential thresholds for the two sexes. We could reach no conclusion when we included other epilepsies or EEG abnormalities in our definition of the trait.

Let us begin with a brief description of what we mean by the polygenic threshold model. Under this model, we hypothesize that there exists some underlying "liability" or susceptibility to the trait. The trait we are interested in here is juvenile myoclonic epilepsy, or JME. We also hypothesize that this liability follows a normal, or Gaussian, distribution.

Biologically, the definition of the polygenic threshold model is as follows: the underlying liability is due to the action of many genetic loci, each with small and equal effects. Moreover, these loci must be additive: that is, there must be no interaction or heterozygosity effects. We emphasize that this is the definition of the polygenic threshold model, and it is actually rather rigorous. The model is *not* a catchall for anything that does not fit a single gene, but rather must fulfill the conditions just mentioned.

We further hypothesize that there exists some threshold or cutoff value, such that individuals with liability greater than this are affected, whereas those whose liability is lower are unaffected (Fig. 1, top).

The model leads to some rather specific predictions about how a polygenic trait will be correlated within families. For example, once an individual is affected, then the mean liability in his/her family is raised, and the frequency of the trait in relatives is increased (Fig. 1, bottom).

[1] Department of Biomathematics and Psychiatry, UCLA School of Medicine. Current address: NY State Psychiatric Institute Columbia University, 722 W. 168th Street, Box 14, New York, NY 10032, USA.

[2] Southwest Regional VA Epilepsy Center, Neurology Service, Wadsworth VA Medical Center, Los Angeles, Current address: Department of Psychiatry, Mt. Sinai medical Center, 1 Gustave Levy Place, New York, NY 10029, USA.

[3] Neurologische Abteilung, Universitätsklinikum Rudolf Virchow, Freie Universität Berlin, Spandauer Damm 130, D-1000 Berlin 19.

[4] Reed Neurological Research Center, UCLA School of Medicine, 710 Westwood Plaza, Los Angeles, CA 90024, USA.

Genetics of the Epilepsies
Beck-Mannagetta et al. (Eds.)

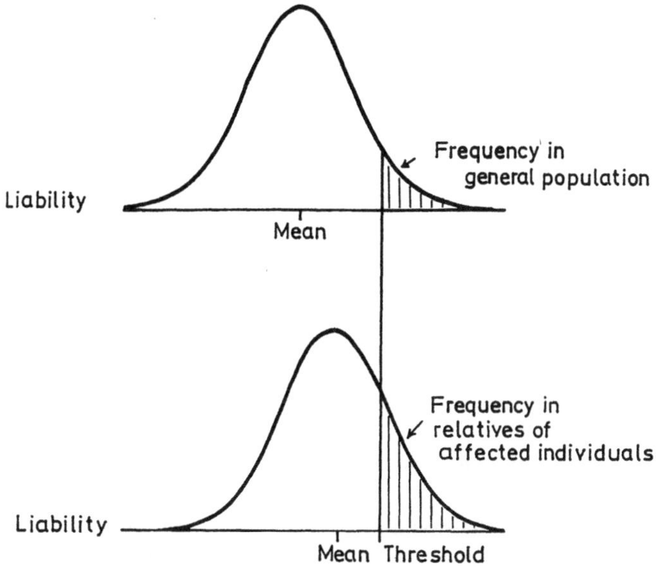

Fig. 1. The polygenic threshold model. Individuals whose liability values fall to the right of the threshold are affected. The *top* graph shows the distribution in the general population. The *bottom* graph shows how the distribution is shifted to the right in the relatives of affected persons

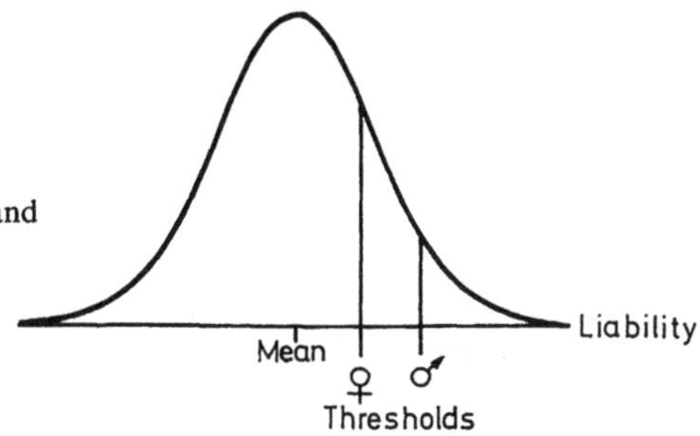

Fig. 2. The polygenic threshold model with differential thresholds for males and females. The graph illustrates the case where females are more frequently affected than males

We can further refine the polygenic threshold model by introducing the idea of differential thresholds for the two sexes (Fig. 2). If females have a lower threshold than males, then we can make additional specific predictions. The first is that, in the general population, more females will be affected than males. The second, less obvious one is that, although males are less often affected, more of the *relatives* of an affected male will be affected than will the relatives of affected females. [In this context we note that in the Tsuboi and Christian data [6] the observed sex ratios go in the opposite direction; that is, females are more often affected than males in the general population, but the relatives of affected females are also more frequently affected than the relatives of affected males (their Table 2). Thus, the Tsuboi and Christian data argue against the polygenic model with differential sex thresholds.]

Table 1. Sex distribution of probands in Berlin and Los Angeles datasets

Probands	Females	Males	Total
Berlin	44	34	78
Los Angeles	20	18	38
	64	52	116

As our first step, we examined the sex distribution of probands in our two datasets: that is, the data collected on families in Berlin [4] and in Los Angeles [2] (Table 1). As the figures reveal, the sex ratio does not deviate significantly from 1 : 1 ($P \cong 0.27$, two-sided). Thus, we abandoned the differential sex model and proceeded to formal analyses of the polygenic threshold model without sex differences.

We actually had three different traits to analyze, i.e., three different ways to define the trait:

1. *Pure JME.* The first and simplest was to define as affected only those individuals who had JME. This represented the narrowest definition.
2. *JME and other epilepsy.* The second definition described as affected all those who had JME or another form of generalized epilepsy; however, families were still ascertained only through pure JME patients.
3. *JME and other epilepsy and EEG abnormalities.* The third and broadest definition included among the affected those with certain defined EEG abnormalities [2], along with the JME and other epilepsy patients as in definition 2.

"Pure" JME was of primary interest, since other authors have speculated that it may be polygenic [3, 6] and the analyses of this turned out to be the most informative, too.

To analyze whether the JME data fit a polygenic model, we used the computer program PGOODFIT [1]. This analysis compares the expected and observed numbers of multiplex families in the dataset. (Multiplex families are those with more than one affected child.) In general, not as many multiplex families are expected under a polygenic model as under single-gene Mendelian inheritance.

The computer program PGOODFIT takes account of family structure (total number of children in the family) and parental status (whether either or both parents are also affected). The user specifies the ascertainment probability (π) and the heritability (h^2). We had *single selection* – that is, each family was ascertained through a single proband – so we set π to 0.001. Since we were interested in the pure polygenic model, we set h^2 to unity. (Actually, the programs were run with h^2 at 0.99, to facilitate convergence.)

Table 2 shows the PGOODFIT results for the three different analyses of 78 Berlin families and 27 Los Angeles families. (There were 38 probands in the Los Angeles dataset, but 11 of those families were not suitable for the PGOODFIT analysis and were therefore not included.)

Under definition 1, "pure JME," the number of multiplex families with JME is on the low side for the polygenic threshold model, although the deviation is not

Table 2. Results of PGOODFIT analyses in Berlin and Los Angeles datasets

Definition	Assumed pop. freq.	No. of multiplex families observed		
		Berlin	Los Angeles	Total
1. Pure JME	0.001	3/78	1/27	4/105*
2. JME + other epilepsy	0.005	8/78	3/27	11/105
3. JME + other epilepsy + EEG abnormalities	0.01	–[a]	7/18	–[a]

* $P \cong 0.06$, two-sided test.
[a] EEGs not done.
Note: None of these results are statistically significant. The P value of ~ 0.06 is the lowest obtained.

statistically significant: $P \cong 0.06$, two-sided test. Remember that a P value of 0.05 would mean we could *reject* the polygenic threshold model. The fact that we have a P value of approximately 0.06 means we cannot formally reject the model, but it does not fit well. (We used the more conservative two-sided test, rather than a one-sided one, because we had no reason a priori to suspect that the number of multiplex families would be too low, as opposed to high, for the polygenic model. Under a one-sided test, the P value would have been approximately 0.03.)

Under definition 2, "JME and other epilepsies," the results were not statistically significant; that is, the observations did not deviate significantly from what is predicted by a polygenic model. For definition 3, which includes the EEG abnormalities found in JME patients as well as in many of their family members, only the Los Angeles dataset contained this information, and then only on 18 families. Again, these observtions did not deviate significantly from what the polygenic model would predict. (The sample size of 18 families for definition 3 was also very small.) This does not mean we have proven that the data do fit a polygenic model – rather, merely that we have no evidence to reject that model for definitions 2 and 3.

It could make sense that JME alone is not polygenic, but that when we include other epilepsies and EEG abnormalities, there may be enough loci involved to look like polygenic inheritance, at least for this rather simple analysis. In particular, Greenberg et al. [2] have shown that, when the EEG abnormalities are included (i.e., under definition 3), the trait may fit a two-locus model of inheritance.

Future Directions

As an overall comment, we can note that each of the two datasets has a particular advantage. The Berlin dataset is relatively large (78 families), whereas the Los Angeles data are rich, in the sense of having information about EEG abnormalities in addition to clinical information about the type of epilepsy. We hope eventually to have EEG data on the Berlin families, too, at which time we will be in a better position to reach more definitive conclusions about the mode of inheritance of JME, both with and without additional forms of epilepsy and both with and without the EEG abnormalities.

In these analyses we examined the fit only with the "pure" polygenic threshold model, that is, with heritability of 1.0 (100%). In this context, heritability represents the proportion of total variance which is due to genetic (as opposed to environmental) factors: $h^2 =$ (genetic variance)/(genetic variance + environmental variance). One could also specify lower heritability values for PGOODFIT and then analyze the corresponding model and its fit with the data.

Also, when we have more data, we may choose to perform a more sophisticated analysis, such as a mixed model, which incorporates a polygenic component, a random environmental component, and a major gene into a single analysis (such as, for example, [5]). Such an analysis would also allow for variable age of onset of JME.

Conclusions

For future directions, therefore, we need to obtain more families for study and to obtain more EEGs on existing families with JME. Until that time, as far as pure polygenic inheritance is concerned, we can only say that, considering JME alone, the polygenic model seems unlikely but is not ruled out definitively; and we cannot conclude anything about JME with other epilepsy, or about JME with other epilepsy and EEG abnormalities, with the data we have available so far.

Acknowledgements. Support for this project was provided by National Institutes of Health grants DK 31813 (S.E.H.), DK 01145 (a Research Career Development Award to S.E.H.), NS 21908 (D.A.G. and A.V.D.-E.), and AM 31775 (D.A.G.), and by the Veterans' Administration.

References

1. Gladstien K, Lange K, Spence MA (1978) A goodness-of-fit test for the polygenic threshold model: application to pyloric stenosis. Am J Med Genet 2:7–13
2. Greenberg DA, Delgado-Escueta AV, Maldonado H, Widelitz H (1987) Segregation analysis of juvenile myoclonic epilepsy (this volume)
3. Janz D (1985) Epilepsy with impulsive petit mal (juvenile myoclonic epilepsy). Acta Neurol Scand 72:449–459
4. Janz D, Durner M, Beck-Mannagetta G, Behl I, Scholz G, Pantazis G (1987) Family studies in juvenile myoclonic epilepsy (this volume)
5. Morton NE, MacLean CJ (1974) Analysis of family resemblance. III. Complex segregation of quantitative traits. Am J Hum Genet 26:489–503
6. Tsuboi T, Christian W (1973) On the genetics of the primary generalized epilepsy with sporadic myclonias of impulsive petit mal type. Humangenetik 19:155–182

Benign Epilepsy of Childhood with Centro-temporal Spikes

S. BLOM [1] and J. HEIJBEL [2]

The Clinical Characteristics, Prevalence, and Rationale

Benign epilepsy in childhood with centro-temporal EEG spikes, also known as benign rolandic epilepsy, is an epileptic syndrome in which the EEG changes are part of the definition. A series of investigations [1–5, 8, 11–13) have shown that the main features are:

1. Partial seizures with symtoms mainly from the orofacial regions. The seizures may become secondarily generalized.
2. The EEG spikes can often be recorded from large areas of the hemisphere, but have a centro-temporal maximum.
3. Both seizures and EEG changes are related to the level of wakefulness. The seizures often occur shortly after the child has gone to sleep and the spikes increase in frequency during drowsiness and sleep. Sometimes they appear during sleep only.
4. The syndrome is uncommon before 3 years of age and has a maximum incidence between 5 and 10 years. The prognosis is good: In most cases the seizures disappear at puberty. The seizures are, with few exceptions, easily controlled with medication. The syndrome has not been observed in adults.

In a prospective incidence study [5], performed in the County of Västerbotten in the Northern part of Sweden, it was found that approximately 25% of epileptic children between the ages 1 and 16 years had benign epilepsy with centro-temporal spikes. The total incidence of childhood epilepsy in the same population was 82/100000. We observed that seizures were sometimes reported both in parents and siblings of the same families. This suggested a hereditary pattern; we therefore decided to perform a genetic study [10]. An autosomal dominant inheritance had been suggested earlier [6]. The investigation was performed in collaboration with Dr. M. Rasmuson at the Department of Genetics, University of Umeå.

Although the seizure description is characteristic, it is not exclusive to this type of epilepsy. We therefore choose the EEG pattern as the genetic marker.

Centro-temporal Spike Pattern

The spikes may be recorded from large areas of the cortex, but are often limited to the central or centro-temporal region only, corresponding to the electrodes C3-

[1] Department of Clinical Neurophysiology, University Hospital, S-75185 Uppsala.
[2] Department of Pediatrics, University Hospital, S-90185 Umcå.

Genetics of the Epilepsies
Beck-Mannagetta et al. (Eds.)

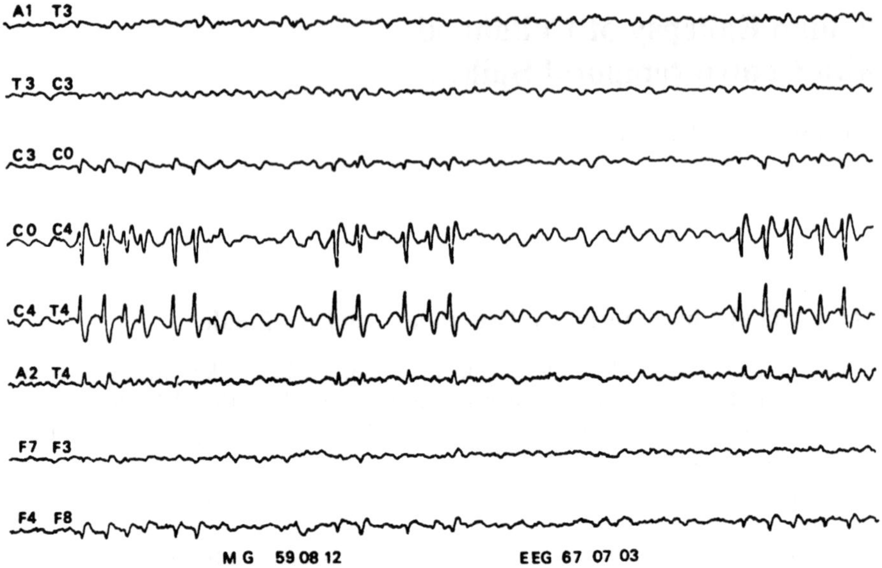

Fig. 1. Interictal EEG recording of 8-year-old boy. He was awake, seizure-free since he was 2 years, on phenobarbital. From [2], by permission

C4 and T3-T4 in the 10–20 system (Fig. 1). The background activity is normal for that age group. The spikes often occur in groups in which the single potentials are identical with respect to duration and amplitude. They may change side at different recordings in the same patient. They increase during sleep and are found only during sleep in some patients.

Lombroso [13] studied the voltage gradient in typical cases. Maximal amplitudes were found pre- and postcentrally and in the midtemporal region. There were fewer high amplitudes in the posterolateral frontal and anterior temporal regions, which is of importance in differentiating rolandic discharges from those found in complex partial epilepsy.

Gregory and Wong [9] recently showed that the greatest positivity is localized frontally, the greatest negativity midtemporally, with the zero crossing in the vicinity of the sylvian fissure. They concluded that a field distribution of this type was probably the result of a horizontally oriented dipole, an unusual finding in clinical electroencephalography. This is important and of further help in identifying cases with benign rolandic epilepsy.

Genetic Study

We selected 19 children as probands from a primary group of about 50 patients. The probands had seizures, the typical EEG changes according to Lombroso's criteria, and at least one sibling between 3 and 13 years of age. The probands were normal to neurological examination, but one of them had a strabismus and another a *vitium organicum cordis*.

The genealogical investigation was performed by means of a personal interview with all parents. Ten probands were boys and 9 girls. Consanguinity was discovered in one family. No geographical cluster was found.

EEGs were recorded for the probands, 32 of 34 siblings (two children below 1 year of age were omitted), and 36 of 38 parents. In one family, the parents refused to take part in the EEG investigation, but denied having had seizures in childhood. The EEG recordings were made during both wakefulness and sleep and included hyperventilation and photic stimulation. In all but three cases a 16-channel EEG machine was used with simultaneous coverage of the frontal, central, and temporal regions. Both bipolar and average reference recordings were obtained.

Figure 2 shows the pedigrees of the investigated families. No parent currently had epilepsy, but four of them (11%) reported seizures during childhood. No information was available regarding the type of seizures for the four parents, and no previous EEG recordings had been performed. In five parents we found a small amount of slow activity in the theta band. Sporadic, low-amplitude centro-temporal spikes were recorded in one of the fathers. This was the first and only time that we observed this in an adult.

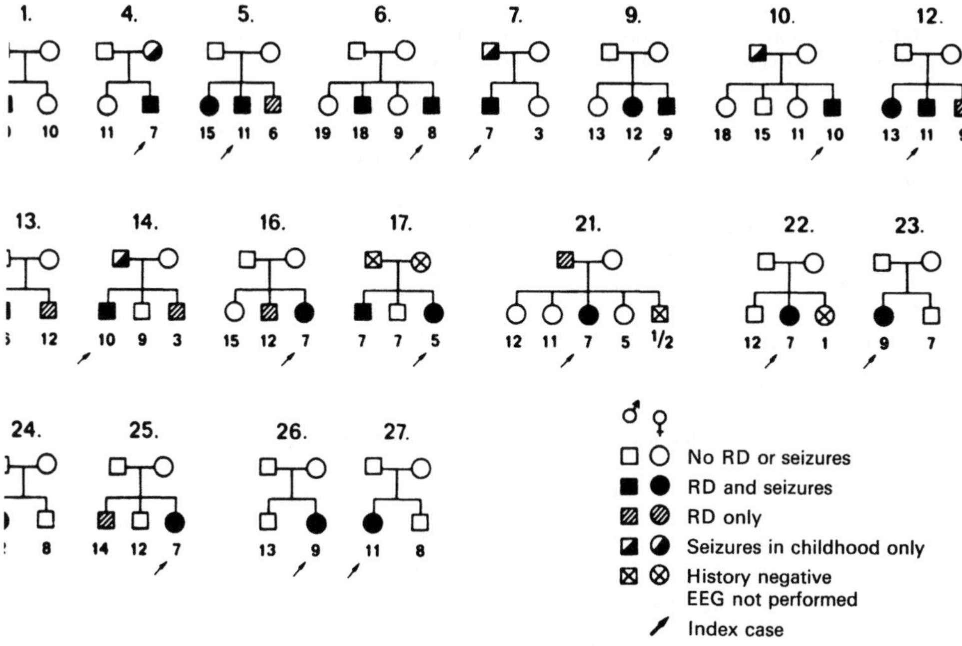

Fig. 2. Pedigrees of 19 families with cases of benign epilepsy in childhood with centro-temporal spikes. Age (years) indicated below each child. RD, Rolandic Discharges. From [10], by permission

Eleven of the siblings (34%) had centro-temporal spikes. Five of these, belonging to five different families, had suffered from seizures. There was no difference in mean age between the children with and the children without seizures. Two of the siblings were slightly mentally retarded, but otherwise no neurological abnormalities were found.

In evaluating the hereditary pattern a sex linkage was ruled out. A recessive mode of inheritance was unlikely, since 4 of 38 parents had seizures during childhood and only one case of consanguinity was discovered. A dominant mode of inheritance was possible. Penetrance may be incomplete, with no clinical history in carriers. In addition, the parents (carriers) had passed the age of clinical and electrophysiological expression. The proportion of affected and unaffected children was tested by using an a priori method: comparing recessive and dominant inheritance patterns (Table 1). When the two children below 1 year of age were excluded and a dominant mode of inheritance was assumed, then there was a close relationship between the expected and the observed number of children with the EEG trait. When a recessive mode of inheritance was tested and the families with one parent with seizures were excluded, a significantly greater number of affected children was found than expected.

Polygenic inheritance was, of course, a possibility and is thought to be of importance in other types of epilepsy with familial occurrence. The number of parents with seizures and the number of affected siblings was, however, considered

Table 1. Analysis by the a priori method of sibships with one or more cases of rolandic discharges (see Fig. 1). From [10], by permission

Size of sibship (n)	No. of sibships (x)	Expected proportion affected (q')	No. affected: Expected ($q'\ n\ x$)	No. affected: Observed
Dominant mode of inheritance, 19 sibships, 51 children. $q = 1/2$				
2	9	2/3	12	10
3	7	4/7	12	16
4	3	8/15	6.4	4
Total	19		30.4	30
$\chi^2_{(1)} = 0.013$	$p > 0.9$			
Recessive mode of inheritance, 14 shibships with symptom-free parents, 36 children. $q = 1/4$				
2	7	4/7	8	8
3	6	16/37	7.8	14
4	1	64/175	1.5	2
Total	14		17.3	24
$\chi^2_{(2)} = 5.07$	p: 0.02–0.03			

q, proportion affected according to the genetic hypothesis.

$q' = \frac{q}{1-(1-q)^n}$, expected proportion of affected children.

to be too high for this mode of inheritance. We did not have an age-matched control group, but in other published reports of healthy children [6, 7] the frequency of children with centro-temporal spikes was 1%–2%, which does not support a polygenic inheritance explanation. Therefore, we concluded that the EEG trait was inherited with an autosomal dominant pattern.

Comments

It is of interest to know whether our criteria for selecting probands resulted in a homogeneous material. It is possible to assess this, at least with respect to the prognosis of EEG changes and seizures. In 1982 we performed a follow-up study of the 40 children with benign epilepsy in childhood [4], first described in 1972 [2]. The aim of the investigation was to study the long-term prognosis. At that time, the probands were adult (mean age 29 years). From the 37 patients identified, we obtained a new history and performed a new EEG recording in 24 cases. One patient abused alcohol and reported occasional seizures of the grand mal type. One woman had been seizure-free for many years but still took medication for fear of loosing her driver's license. All other patients had been seizure-free for many years, were off medication, and had normal EEGs. These findings indicate that the material was homogeneous. Further genetic studies of benign epilepsy in childhood with centro-temporal spikes should, however, also consider the following points:

1. The seizure types and the EEG changes of the parents should be studied in detail.
2. The offspring of the probands should be investigated clinically and with EEG.
3. The EEG marker, the centro-temporal spike, should fulfill the criteria of Gregory and Wong [12] with regard to field distribution.
4. Biochemical variables that could be related to the epilepsy should be searched for.

References

1. Beaussart M (1972) Benign epilepsy of children with rolandic (centro-temporal) paroxysmal foci. Epilepsia 13:795–811
2. Blom S, Heijbel J, Bergfors PG (1972) Benign epilepsy of children with centro-temporal EEG foci – prevalence and follow-up study of 40 patients. Epilepsia 13:609–619
3. Blom S, Heijbel J (1975) Benign epilepsy of childhood with centrotemporal EEG foci – discharge rate during sleep. Epilepsia 16:133–140
4. Blom S, Heijbel J, Bergfors PG (1978) Incidence of epilepsy in children: a follow-up study three years after the first seizure. Epilepsia 19:343–350
5. Blom S, Heijbel J (1982) Begnign epilepsy of children with centrotemporal EEG foci: a follow-up study in adulthood of patients initially studied as children. Epilepsia 23:629–631
6. Bray PF, Wiser WC (1965) Hereditary characteristics of familial temporal-central focal epilepsy. Pediatrics 36:207–211
7. Eeg-Olofsson O, Petersen I, Sellden U (1971) The development of the electroencephalogram in normal children from the age of 1 through 15 years. Paroxysmal activity. Neuropädiatrie 4:375–404

8. Gibbs EL, Gibbs FA (1959–1960) Good prognosis of mid-temporal epilepsy. Epilepsia 1:448–453
9. Gregory DL, Wong PK (1984) Topographical analysis of the centrotemporal discharges in benign Rolandic epilepsy of childhood. Epilepsia 25:705–711
10. Heijbel J, Blom S, Rasmuson M (1975) Benign epilepsy of childhood with centrotemporal EEG foci: a genetic study. Epilepsia 16:285–293
11. Lerman P, Kivity S (1975) Benign focal epilepsy of childhood – a follow up study of 100 recovered patients. Arch Neurol 32:261–264
12. Loiseau P, Beaussart M (1973) The seizures of benign childhood epilepsy with rolandic paroxysmal discharges. Epilepsia 14:381–389
13. Lombroso CT (1967) Sylvian seizures and mid-temporal spike foci in children. Arch Neurol 17:52–59

Genetics of the Partial Epilepsies

D. M. TREIMAN [1]

In the proposed international classification of epilepsies [8], epilepsy syndromes are divided into those which are generalized and those which are localization related. Within each of these categories a further distinction is made between those epilepsy syndromes which are idiopathic and those which are symptomatic. In this classification scheme the implication of the term idiopathic is that the disorder is a primary one, that is, intrinsic to the individual and not secondary to some acquired insult. Thus, in this approach to classification the term idiopathic is synonymous with the term genetic or hereditary. There is, in fact, abundant evidence for a genetic etiology in the idiopathic epilepsy syndromes, a number of which are discussed in this volume.

Most people with epilepsy, however, suffer from one of the acquired partial onset epilepsy syndromes and the evidence for a genetic component in the etiology of these syndromes is far less clear. Table 1 presents the frequencies of generalized and partial onset epilepsies in children and adults when data from four

[1] Department of Neurology, Reed Neurological Research Center, UCLA School of Medicine, 710 Westwood Plaza, Los Angeles, CA 90024, USA.

Table 1. Relative frequencies of types of epilepsy. After Treiman [38]

	Children (%)	Adults (%)
Total number of cases	4159	4751
Unclassifiable	24.5	13.2
Generalized epilepsies	34.4	19.7
Primary generalized	22.9	18.0
"grand mal"	6.8	11.3
"petit mal"	10.4	2.5
myoclonic	2.2	3.8
other	3.5	0.6
Secondary generalized	11.5	1.6
Lennox-Gastaut syndrome	7.1	0.9
infantile spasms	1.9	0.0
other	2.5	0.7
Partial epilepsies	40.1	67.1
With elementary symptomatology (focal)	13.6	15.2
With complex symptomatology (psychomotor)	14.0	41.4
With secondarily generalized seizures	12.5	10.5

Genetics of the Epilepsies
Beck-Mannagetta et al. (Eds.)

large studies [2, 3, 15, 24] were combined [38]. Partial onset epilepsies, almost all of which were symptomatic in these patients, accounted for about 70% of the adult patients with epilepsy and about 40% of the children with epilepsy. In most series a specific etiology has been identified in about two-thirds of the patients [30] on the basis of clinical signs and symptoms. Cortical pathology has been seen on examination of most neurosurgical specimens acquired at the time of cortical resection for control of intractable partial epilepsy [7, 14, 18].

However, not all patients who suffer cerebral cortical insults develop epilepsy. Even in patients who have suffered a depressed skull fracture or intracranial hematoma as the result of severe head injuries, the incidence of epilepsy following such head trauma is only around 25% [22].

Rimoin and Metrakos [34] studied the incidence of seizures in families of children with infantile hemiplegia. Seizures occurred more frequently in families with children who had hemiplegia and seizures than in control families. In comparison with control families, however, the incidence of family history for seizures was lower in the families of those children with hemiplegia who did not develop seizures. Similar data have been reported for cerebral tumors and for post-traumatic epilepsy. The incidence of epilepsy in families of patients with tumors and epilepsy is higher (7%) than in the families of patients with cerebral tumors who do not develop epilepsy (2%) [25, 29].

Identical findings have been observed in head injury patients. Four hundred twenty-two American servicemen who sustained head injuries during the Korean War were studied. Eighty-three experienced one seizure more than 1 month after injury. Seven percent of the seizure patients and 2% of the nonseizures head injury patients had a family history positive for epilepsy [13].

These data suggest that there must be factors which make some patients more susceptible to the development of epilepsy following cerebral insult and other factors which may confer resistance to the development of epilepsy. It is likely that such epilepsy susceptibility or epilepsy resistance factors are transmitted genetically. If this is the case, then there should be a greater occurrence of epilepsy in affected families than would be expected by chance.

This chapter will review those studies which have attempted to ascertain whether or not there is a familial component in the etiology of acquired partial onset epilepsies, summarize what is known about the mechanism whereby such hereditary factors might be operant, and indicate what directions future research should take in the consideration of a genetic role in the etiology of partial onset seizures.

Previous Studies

A number of studies have evaluated the incidence of positive family history in patients with partial onset seizures. Lennox [26] divided 4231 epileptic patients into two types, symptomatic and idiopathic, and studied 20000 of their relatives. The prevalence of epilepsy in near relatives of those in the idiopathic group was 3.6% whereas the prevalence for the symptomatic group was 1.8%. He compared these figures to the prevalence rate of 0.5% reported for draftees into the U.S. Armed

Services during World Wars I and II. At about the same time Alström [1] reported a study of 897 epileptics. He found the mean prevalence of epilepsy among their first degree relatives was 1.5%. The prevalence was highest in relatives of patients with epilepsy of unknown etiology. Harvald [19] studied 237 Danish patients and found the prevalence of epilepsy among near relatives of patients with idiopathic epilepsy was 4.2%, compared with 2.6% for all of the relatives of the 237 patients and 0.46% in the population of Denmark at that time. Smith et al. [36] reviewed clinical records from 2090 epileptic children and adult patients. The data for 1648 of them were adequate for analysis. Of these, 535 were believed to have evidence of a neuropathologic lesion that antedated the first seizure and thus most likely had symptomatic partial onset epilepsy. Twenty-four percent of these patients had a family history of epilepsy. For comparison, these authors cited data from a control group of hospital personnel numbering 722, where only 6.6% of the hospital personnel reported known epilepsy among relatives [37].

Holowach et al. [20] studied 114 cases of Jacksonian epilepsy in infants and children seen at the St. Louis Children's Hospital from 1934 to 1954 or at the Pediatric Convulsive Clinic from 1950 to 1955. Family history information was available for 95 of the children. The family history was positive in 27 cases (28%). In half of the cases, epilepsy was present in either the parents or siblings. In another series from the same institution, Holowach et al. [21] reviewed psychomotor epilepsy in 120 children. Family history was available in 100 of the cases and was positive for epilepsy in 55 cases. The incidence of positive family history in first degree relatives (parents and siblings) was 23%. Currie et al. [9] studied 666 patients with temporal lobe epilepsy. Seventy-three (11%) had a family history of epilepsy in one or more close relatives. No control group was studied.

Gerken et al. [16] studied 203 epileptic children who had demonstrated at least one focal sharp wave on the EEG. Twenty-three percent had a positive family history for epilepsy, in contrast to 30% of children with spike-wave absences [11] and 6% in a control group [10]. In 150 of the probands sufficient data were available to determine the percentage of relatives at risk. Of such relatives, 2.5% had epilepsy in contrast to 4.4% of the relatives of patients with spike-wave absences [11]. In both groups, mothers and their siblings were more often affected than fathers and their siblings. Sixty percent of the 203 probands and 18% of their siblings showed "centrencephalic" EEG patterns [12]. These authors suggested that genetically determined seizure susceptibility plays an important role in the pathogenesis of epilepsy with focal sharp waves.

The higher prevalence of epilepsy in the probands' mothers and the mothers' siblings has also been observed by others. Annegers et al. [5] studied 908 children with one epileptic parent. A higher than expected number of children whose mothers had epilepsy also suffered from seizures (epilepsy or febrile convulsions), whereas no such increase was detected among the children of affected fathers.

A number of investigators have studied possible genetic factors in patients with medically intractable partial onset epilepsy who have undergone surgical procedures for control of their seizures. Penfield and Paine [32] reviewed the 234 patients with intractable epilepsy who had undergone craniotomy for removal of the seizure focus by Penfield at the Montreal Neurological Institute during the 6-year period from 1945 through 1950. All but ten had data available regarding family history. Ten of the 224 patients studied (4.4%) had near relatives with epilepsy. More distant relatives of an additional seven patients had had one or more convulsion. Because the average number of near relatives, calculated from the Canadian census figures, was about five for each patient, Penfield and Paine calculated that the prevalence of epilepsy in the total number of near relatives in this series was below 1%. Thus they concluded there was no evidence for a genetic component in the etiology of the focal epilepsy in their group of 224 patients treated surgically.

In another study of the occurrence of epilepsy in the families of patients with focal epilepsy treated surgically at the Montreal Neurological Institute, Andermann [4] and her colleagues evaluated 60 patients. They found a prevalence of one or more seizures in first degree relatives of 3.5%. This was only slightly higher than the prevalence in a control group of 2.9%. The highest incidence was found in the siblings and the offspring of both probands and controls.

Falconer et al. [14] reviewed the genetic and etiologic factors in temporal lobe epilepsy in two slightly overlapping series of 100 consecutive patients treated surgically. Of those with mesial temporal sclerosis or miscellaneous scars and infarcts, 13%–20% had a positive family history of epilepsy in first degree relatives. Twenty-three percent of the first series and 17% of the second series had a history of prolonged febrile convulsions. Falconer proposed a relationship between prolonged febrile convulsions and a positive family history for epilepsy and suggested that "the inherited factor probably acts by predisposing the infant to epilepsy once it develops fever. The nerve cell damage then substained as a result of hypoxia in time develops into an epileptogenic lesion in its own right."

Lindsay [28] also suggested a relationship between the occurrence of febrile seizures and a genetic susceptibility to the development of epilepsy. She studied 99 children with temporal lobe epilepsy. The 99 probands had 214 siblings, 32 of whom had definite convulsive disorders. Thus the uncorrected prevalence of seizure disorders in the siblings was 15%, a figure much in excess of the prevalence found in the general population. When the 99 children were divided into three groups the risk of epilepsy among brothers and sisters of children who had sustained a severe cerebral insult was 1.9%. The risk of a positive history for epilepsy among siblings in those probands who had sustained at least one episode of status epilepticus was 30%. The risk to the siblings of probands who had neither an episode of severe cerebral insult nor status epilepticus was 9%. Twenty-four of the 32 affected siblings of probands had febrile convulsions. Twenty of the 24 of those with a history of febrile convulsions were the siblings of the probands with status epilepticus. On the basis of these data, Lindsay suggested that the susceptibility to convulsions in the presence of fever is inherited and that prolonged febrile convulsions, at least in some cases, leads to the development of mesial temporal sclerosis and chronic epilepsy. Thus, Lindsey suggested that a higher prevalence of temporal lobe epilepsy among siblings of probands than would be predicted by chance might be explained by the occurrence of a genetic susceptibility to convulsions in the presence of fever.

Jensen [23] also reviewed genetic factors in temporal lobe epilepsy in a group of patients who underwent unilateral temporolobectomy. She studied 74 patients. Twenty-two (29.7%) had a family history of epilepsy afflicting 38 relatives. The

74 patients had a total of 171 siblings and of these five siblings of four patients had epilepsy. This results in a prevalence of epilepsy among siblings of 2.9% for this series.

Several studies have looked at the incidence of epilepsy in twins in order to evaluate a possible genetic component to the epilepsy. Lennox and Lennox [27] studied 121 pairs with cryptogenic epilepsy. Thirteen of these pairs were monozygotic twins with temporal lobe seizures. Five of the 13 pairs (38%) were concordant with regard to the type of seizure. In 51 twin pairs with generalized tonic-clonic seizures there was concordance in 82%, and in 20 pairs with petit mal epilepsy there was concordance in 75% of the cases. Barslund and Danielsen [6] studied three families in which cryptogenic temporal lobe epilepsy was present in monozygotic twins. There was no evidence of birth injury in any of the twin pairs although one mother had hemoptysis during pregnancy and possibly slight toxemia of pregnancy. In all three families temporal lobe spike foci were found in the near relatives of the twins or there were reports of epileptic seizures in near relatives.

The data cited above suggest that there is a greater incidence of positive family history for epilepsy in patients with partial onset seizures than might be expected by chance, but that this incidence is less than that observed in families of patients with primary generalized idiopathic seizure disorders. However, a number of the studies included patients with mixed seizure types or poorly defined seizure types, and many included both children and adults in the same series. Some of the studies suggested that there is no genetic component in the etiology of symptomatic adult onset partial epilepsy.

VA Cooperative Study

In order to ascertain whether there is a genetically transmitted susceptibility to epilepsy in adult onset partial epilepsies and to determine what factors might be associated with or predictive of such positive family histories, family history data [39] were collected from a group of partial onset seizure patients participating in a prospective randomized clinical trial of antiepileptic drugs in the treatment of newly diagnosed seizure disorders in adults.

The study was carried out as part of a ten hospital, nationwide Veteran's Administration cooperative study to determine the best treatment of new onset seizure disorders in adults [30]. Newly diagnosed or clearly subtherapeutic patients aged 18 to 70 were classified into one of three groups depending on which partial seizure type was most prominent in the individual patient: secondarily generalized tonic-clonic, complex partial, and simple partial. The patients were then randomly assigned to one of the following drugs: phenobarbital, phenytoin, primidone, or carbamazepine. A detailed seizure history, medical history, and family history were obtained prior to randomization; an EEG was also recorded prior to randomization. The history, including a detailed family history, was reviewed after 2 years and at the end of the study. All of the family history data was obtained from the patient by historical reporting and was not independently verified.

The study population consisted of 612 patients. Eighty-seven percent were males and 90% were veterans of the United States armed services. The mean age was 41 years, mean I.Q. 100, and mean education 13 years. Three hundred fifty-one patients were assigned to the secondarily generalized tonic-clonic group, 200 to the complex partial seizure group, and 61 to the simple partial seizure group. Seizure etiology was determined in two-thirds of the cases. Trauma caused the seizure disorder in 34% and cerebral vascular disorder in 14%, a variety of other causes accounted for 18%. Thirty-four percent were unknown.

One hundred fifty-one of 612 patients (27.7%) with partial seizures had one or more first or second degree relatives with seizures. Fifty-two of the 612 patients (9.2%) with partial seizures had one or more siblings with seizures.

In order to evaluate the association of various historical and EEG factors with positive family history, a contingency table was constructed for each factor. Chi square analysis for statistical significance was performed for each factor. The results of this analysis are presented in Table 2. These results suggest the existence of possible hereditary factors in partial seizure patients. Table 3 lists factors which were not significantly correlated with positive family history.

In order to identify factors predictive of a positive family history for seizures which could be utilized in a meaningful way (i.e., for genetic counseling), the data were reanalyzed using only a history of seizures in siblings as the criterion for

Table 2. Historical and EEG factors positively and negatively correlated with positive family history

	χ^2	P
Positively correlated		
Age at onset <21 years	34.9	<0.001
History of febrile seizures	23.1	<0.001
Polyspike waves on EEG	7.9	<0.05
Female sex	35.1	<0.001
Negatively Correlated		
Postinfarction etiology	13.0	<0.005

Table 3. Factors not significantly correlated with positive family history

Race
Abnormal EEG
Sharp waves on EEG
Spike-wave discharges on EEG
Polyspike discharges on EEG
Congenital etiology
Postalcohol etiology
Posttraumatic etiology
Spike discharges on EEG
Seizure type

Table 4. Factors positively and negatively correlated with positive family history in siblings

	χ^2	P
Positively correlated		
Age of onset <21 years	4.0	<0.05
Female sex	4.0	<0.05
Parent with seizures	39.0	<0.001
2nd or 3nd degree relative with seizures	14.4	<0.001
Negatively correlated		
Postinfarction etiology	4.9	<0.05

positive family history. Table 4 presents factors significantly correlated with positive family history in siblings on chi square analysis.

The finding that "parents with seizures" and "second or third degree relatives with seizures" are predictors of the probability of seizures in siblings suggests a familial and possibly genetic role in the etiology of seizures in this population of partial onset seizure patients.

Summary and Conclusions

The data from the studies discussed above, including the VA cooperative study, suggest that there is a small but real increase in the incidence of epilepsy in family members of patients with partial onset seizures. Clearly, acquired partial onset seizures are not inherited in a Mendelian fashion, as may be the case with some of the primary generalized childhood onset epilepsies discussed elsewhere in this volume. It appears, rather, that the increased incidence of positive family histories in families of patients with partial onset seizures can be best explained by the inheritance of a greater susceptibility to epilepsy in the presence of other cerebral insults.

The mechanism whereby such susceptibility is mediated is not yet known. However, several theories are worth consideration. The occurrence of prolonged febrile convulsions has been suggested by a number of authors as at least one of the causative factors of mesial temporal sclerosis. If there is an inherited susceptibility to prolonged convulsions in the presence of fever, this might be an explanation for an increased incidence of temporal lobe epilepsy occurring in the same family if the febrile seizure hypothesis is valid.

Gloor [17] has suggested that patients with primary generalized epilepsies have an abnormality of neuronal membranes which is generalized and found in all neurons. It may be that some patients have such an abnormality of sufficient degree that their seizures are manifested as primary generalized epilepsies with childhood onset. There may be other patients who have some degree of neuronal membrane alteration, not sufficient to give rise to spontaneous idiopathic primary generalized epilepsies, but sufficient so that when such neurons are subjected to insult they become epileptic. The exact abnormality present in such neurons, if one exists, has not yet been ascertained. However, only relatively small changes in the function of various ion channels or in the number or function of excitatory or inhibitory amino acid receptors would be necessary to allow the development of a seizure focus. Prince [33] has pointed out that only a 9% suppression of GABA mediated synaptic inhibition by bicuculline is necessary to generate epileptiform events in rat neocortical tissue slices.

Epileptic susceptibility, however, might not be related to neuronal structure or function but rather to alterations in the extent of glial cell proliferation, which may occur in response to cortical injury. Small alterations in the number of glial cells which invade a cortical scar may have significant impact on the amount of extracellular potassium available in the neuronal extracellular environment. Relatively small changes in the amount of extracellular potassium may result in the development of spontaneous epileptic activity in a focus of cortical injury.

It may be that susceptibility to the development of seizure disorders following cerebral insult is not due to any genetic difference in neuronal or glial structure or function but rather to genetic differences in extracerebral factors. Panter et al. [31] have reported intriguing data on genetic differences in serum haptoglobin levels and have suggested that such differences may account for certain forms of familial epilepsy because of the role haptoglobin plays in clearing iron from an injury site. There is considerable evidence that iron compounds play a role in the pathogenesis of CNS damage. Epileptiform seizures and EEG abnormalities can be experimentally produced by the intercerebral injection of either iron solids or hemoglobin [35, 40].

Directions of Future Research

If epilepsy susceptibility factors can be identified, this should open the way to the development of therapeutic interventions which could prevent the development of epilepsy when such susceptibility carriers are exposed to cerebral insult. By identifying families in which there is an increased susceptibility to epilepsy, it may be possible to identify such factors. As human gene maps are expanded it will be possible to study the inheritance of factors such as haptoglobin which may play a role in the susceptibility to epilepsy following cerebral trauma. It may also be possible to identify some families with acquired epilepsy in enough of the family members to do DNA polymorphism studies, such as those described elsewhere in this volume, and thus localize an epilepsy susceptibility gene. As the pathophysiology of cortical epilepsy becomes better understood – especially in terms of neurotransmitters, ion channels, and amino acid receptors – it should be possible to use candidate genes to screen such families directly for specific alterations in neuronal or glial function which may underlie a genetic susceptibility to epilepsy after cortical insult. This, in turn, may lead to techniques for the prevention of cortical epilepsy following cerebral insult and thus to a significant reduction in the incidence of the acquired epilepsies.

References

1. Alström CH (1950) A study of epilepsy in its clinical, social and genetic aspects. Acta Psychiatr Neurol Suppl 63:1–284
2. Alving J (1978) Classification of the epilepsies: an investigation of 1508 consecutive adult patients. Acta Neurol Scand 58:205–212
3. Alving J (1979) Classification of the epilepsies: an investigation of 402 children. Acta Neurol Scand 60:157–163
4. Andermann E (1982) Multifactorial inheritance of generalized and focal epilepsy. In: Anderson VE, Hauser WA, Penry JK, Sing CF (eds) Genetic basis of the epilepsies. Raven, New York, pp 355–374
5. Annegers JF, Hauser WA, Elveback LR, Anderson VE, Kurland LT (1976) Seizure disorders in offspring of parents with a history of seizures – a maternal-paternal difference? Epilepsia 17:1–9
6. Barslund I, Danielsen J (1963) Temporal epilepsy in monozygotic twins. Epilepsia 4:138–150

7. Brown JD (1973) Structural substrates of seizure foci in the human temporal lobe. UCLA Forum in Medical Sciences 17:339–374
8. Commission on Classification and Terminology of the International League Against Epilepsy (1985) Proposal for classification of epilepsies and epileptic syndromes. Epilepsia 26:268–278
9. Currie S, Healthfield KWG, Henson RA, Scott DF (1971) Clinical course and prognosis of temporal lobe epilepsy. A survey of 666 patients. Brain 94:173–190
10. Doose H, Gerken H, Hien-Völpel KF, Völzke E (1969) Genetics of photosensitive epilepsy. Neuropädiatrie 1:56–73
11. Doose H, Gerken H, Horstmann T, Völzke E (1973) Genetic factors in spike-wave absences. Epilepsia 14:57–75
12. Doose H, Gerken H, Kiefer R, Völzke E (1977) Genetic factors in childhood epilepsy with focal sharp waves. II. EEG findings in patients and siblings. Neuropädiatrie 8:10–20
13. Evans JH (1962) Post-traumatic epilepsy. Neurology 12:665–674
14. Falconer MA (1971) Genetic and related aetiological factors in temporal lobe epilepsy. A review. Epilepsia 12:13–31
15. Gastaut H, Gastaut JL, Goncalves e Silva GE, Fernandez Sanchez GR (1975) Relative frequency of different types of epilepsy: a study employing the classification of the International League Against Epilepsy. Epilepsia 16:457–461
16. Gerken H, Kiefer R, Doose H, Völzke (1977) Genetic factors in childhood epilepsy with focal sharp waves. I. Clinical data and familial morbidity for seizures. Neuropädiatrie 8:3–9
17. Gloor P (1979) Generalized epilepsy with spike-and-wave discharge; a reinterpretation of its electroencephalographic and clinical manifestations. The 1977 William G. Lennox Lecture, American Epilepsy Society. Epilepsia 20:571–588
18. Green JR, Scheetz DG (1964) Surgery of epileptogenic lesions of the temporal lobe. Arch Neurol 10:135–148
19. Harvald B (1954) Heredity in epilepsy: an electroencephalographic study of relatives of epileptics. Enjar Munksgaard, Copenhagen
20. Holowach J, Thursten DL, O'Leary J (1958) Jacksonian seizures in infancy and childhood. J Pediat 52:670–686
21. Holowach J, Renda YA, Wapner J (1961) Psychomotor seizures in childhood. J Pediat 59:339–346
22. Jennett B (1982) Post-traumatic epilepsy. In: Laidlaw J, Richen A (eds) A textbook of epilepsy. Churchill Livingstone, New York, pp 146–154
23. Jensen I (1975) Genetic factors in temporal lobe epilepsy. Acta Neurol Scand 52:381–394
24. Joshi V, Katiyar BC, Mohan PK, Misra S, Shukla GD (1977) Profile of epilepsy in a developing country: a study of 1000 patients based on the international classification. Epilepsia 18:549–553
25. Kirstein L (1942) Epilepsie bei intrakraniellen expansiven Prozessen. Acta Neurol Scand 50:12–20
26. Lennox WG (1951) Heredity of epilepsy as told by relatives and twins. JAMA 146:529–536
27. Lennox WG, Lennox MA (1960) Epilepsy and related disorders. Churchill, London
28. Lindsay JMM (1971) Genetics and epilepsy: A model from critical path analysis. Epilepsia 12:47–54
29. Lund M (1952) Epilepsy in association with intracranial tumor. Acta Psychiatr Neurol Scand Suppl 81:3–149
30. Mattson RH, Cramer JA, Collins JF, Smith DB, Delgado-Escueta AV, Browne TR, Williamson PD, Treiman DM, McNamara JO, McCutchen CB, Homan RW, Crill WE, Lubozynski MF, Rosenthal NP, Mayersdorf A (1985) Comparison of carbamazepine, phenobarbital, phenytoin, and primidone in partial and secondarily generalized tonic-clonic seizures. N Engl J Med 313:145–151
31. Panter SS, Sadrzadeh MH, Hallaway PE, Haines JL, Eaton JW (1985) Hypohaptoglobinemia: association with familial epilepsy. J Exp Med 161:748–754
32. Penfield W, Paine K (1955) Results of surgical therapy for focal epileptic seizures. Can Med Assoc J 73:515–531
33. Prince DA (1987) Epilepsy in a dish: an old recipe with new sauces. The 1987 William G. Lennox Lecture, American Epilepsy Society. December 8, 1987

34. Rimoin DL, Metrakos JD (1963) The genetics of convulsive disorders in the families of hemiplegics. In: Mendel G (ed) Proc II Intern Congr Hum Genet pp 1655–1658
35. Rosen AD, Frumin NV (1979) Focal epileptogenesis after intracortical hemoglobin injection. Exp Neurol 66:227–284
36. Smith BS, Robinson GC, Lennox WG (1954) Acquired epilepsy. A study of 535 cases. Neurology 4:19–28
37. Stein C (1933) Hereditary factors in epilepsy. Am J Psychiatr 89:989–1037
38. Treiman D (1981) Seizure types and causes of epilepsy. Seminars in Neurology 1:65–75
39. Treiman D and the VA Epilepsy Cooperative Study Group. Evidence for hereditary factors in adult onset partial seizures (to be submitted to Epilepsia)
40. Willmore LJ, Sypert GW, Munson JB, Hurd RW (1978) Chronic focal epileptiform discharges induced by injection of iron into rat and cat cortex. Science 200:1501–1503

Genetics of EEG-Characteristics

Genetic Variation of the Normal Human EEG

F. Vogel [1]

Since the EEG plays a key role in the diagnosis and classification of epilepsies, and since it shows an appreciable variability in the "normal" range, the question as to the causes of this "normal" variability might be of interest for our understanding of epilepsy. It is well-known that external influences (such as sensory input), changes in the chemical parameters of the blood (such as decrease of CO_2 level, hypoglycemia, or altered metabolite levels due to malfunction of the liver) may lead to transitory or even long lasting modifications of the EEG (see [2]). Here, the EEG indicates an abnormal state of brain function. But even under normal conditions in individuals who are awake, relaxed, and resting with closed eyes, there is still appreciable interindividual variability, whereas the EEG of the same individual remains practically constant even over long time periods. Characteristic changes occur both during childhood and youth, and with adults of advancing age. This interindividual variability of the resting EEG in the normal range is largely genetically determined, as has been shown by studies on monozygotic (MZ) twins (for the older literature see [16]; for reviews see [19, 20]:

1. Resting EEGs of healthy MZ twins are as similar as consecutive EEG records from the same individual under constant conditions (Fig. 1). This impression is corroborated by computerized quantitative EEG analysis [15].
2. Even MZ twins separated in infancy or childhood show very similar [7] or practically identical [9] EEG records.
3. Speed of EEG maturation during childhood and youth also shows genetic variability, as indicated by the EEG similarity in MZ twins in contrast to otherwise considerable interindividual variability.
4. Of the well-known EEG changes in advanced age, slowing of the alpha rhythm, decrease in amplitude, or increase in theta activity in the anterior leads are concordant in MZ twins. On the other hand, discordances in mild anomalies, such as temporal focal abnormalities or short bursts of bilaterally synchronous theta waves, are common [6].
5. Discordance in neurotic symptoms of MZ twins does not lead to a discordant EEG [23].

[1] Institut für Humangenetik und Anthropologie, Universität Heidelberg, Im Neuenheimer Feld 328, D-6900 Heidelberg.

Genetics of the Epilepsies
Beck-Mannagetta et al. (Eds.)

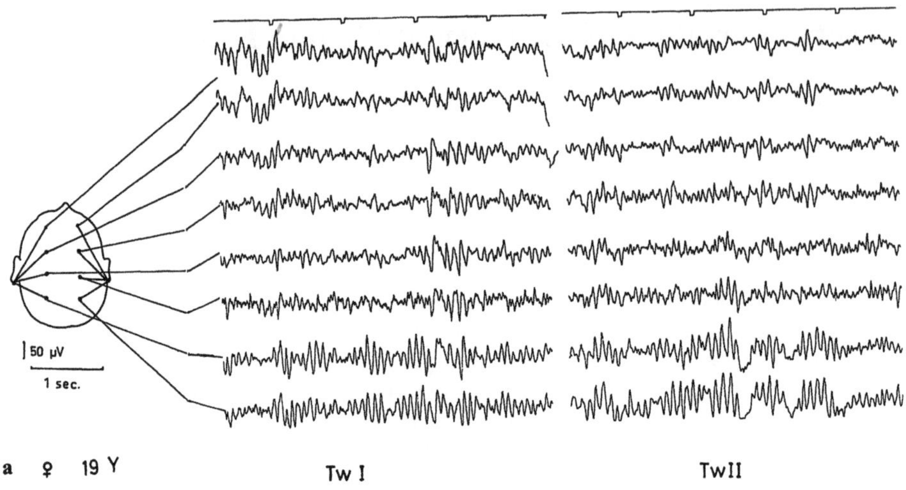

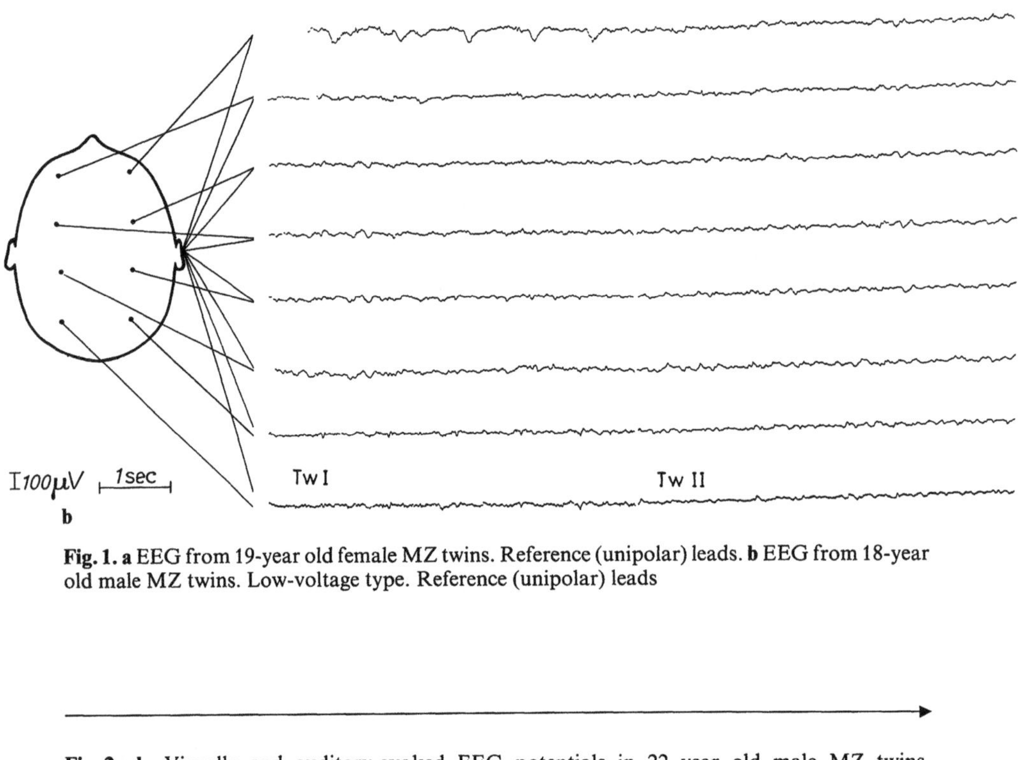

Fig. 1. a EEG from 19-year old female MZ twins. Reference (unipolar) leads. **b** EEG from 18-year old male MZ twins. Low-voltage type. Reference (unipolar) leads

Fig. 2a, b. Visually and auditory-evoked EEG potentials in 22 year old male MZ twins. Electrode: Cz. **a** Visually evoked potentials in four intensity levels (*1*, lowest intensity; *4*, highest intensity; stimulation with 64 flashes each in pseudo-randomized order, 256 flashes altogether. Stimulation with closed eyes). **b** *5*, Auditory-evoked potentials; 256 acoustic stimuli; stimulation with closed eyes. Tw I ———; Tw II – – – –. (For details of the experimental setup, see [24].)

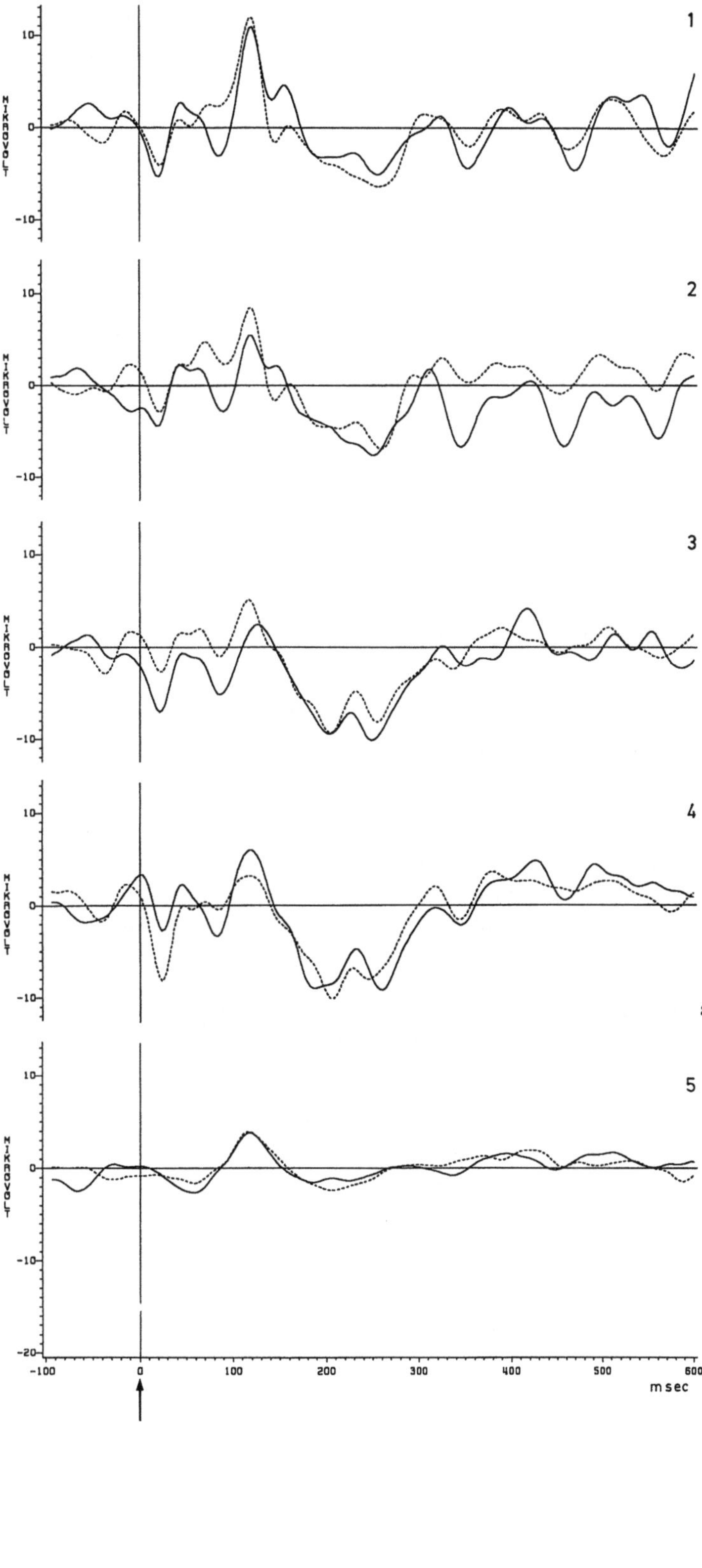

a

b

6. EEG changes under controlled external and experimental conditions, such as during nocturnal sleep [16, 26], EEG synchronization under hyperventilation, and alcohol ingestion [12], are under genetic control.
7. High concordance in MZ twins has also been described for visually and auditory-evoked EEG potentials [3, 1] (Fig. 2).

Ever since the early days of EEG research, family studies have been performed very often. Studies on EEG abnormalities or „borderline" records, found among close relatives of epileptic patients more frequently than in the general population, are discussed in other contributions in this volume. Here, we shall confine ourselves to EEG variation observed within the normal range and without known relationship to disease liabilities.

Whereas twin studies can help to answer the very general question to what degree variability in a certain phenotype has a genetic basis, family studies may point to more specific genetic mechanisms. In view of the multidimensional complexity of EEG variation, however, such studies promise deeper insights only if relatively distinct EEG variants are investigated. Such variants exist.

Family Studies on Variants of Alpha Activity (Fig. 3–6)

The most striking alpha variant is the low-voltage EEG, which occurs in about 4% of our adult population and which manifests itself during the second decade of life (Fig. 3). There is an almost completely bimodal distribution of alpha activity as measured by the alpha index within families, and the segregation ratios point to a monogenic and autosomal dominant mode of inheritance ([2, 17], see also [19]). Another variant of the alpha rhythm is characterized by almost sinusoid, monomorphic alpha waves in all unipolar leads (Fig. 4). This was also found in about 4% of the adult population [21]. Even within families, this alpha rhythm cannot be distinguished quite as easily from more average EEG characteristics as the low-voltage type, but family studies have also pointed to the presence of a major gene with an autosomal dominant mode of inheritance.

In a third, and much rarer variant (~0.6%), alpha waves are replaced by occipital 16–19 cycle/s waves, which are blocked like alpha waves when the eyes are opened (Fig. 5). After closing of the eyes, alpha waves may appear for a few seconds, soon to be replaced, however, by 16–19 cycle/s waves. Studies in eight families showed a simple autosomal dominant mode of inheritance.

Another rare EEG variant has found much attention: the 4–5 cycle/s rhythm (Fig. 6). The resting EEG shows relatively regular 4–5 cycle/s waves, mostly with occipital or occipitotemporal localizations. This rhythm can be easily disturbed by sensory stimuli; the 4–5 cycle/s waves are then replaced by alpha waves for a short time. The 4–5 cycle/s waves also disappear when the eyes are opened; after closing the eyes, they reappear after a short sequence of alpha waves. This trait is found in about 1‰ of healthy adult individuals. The fact that the subjects car-

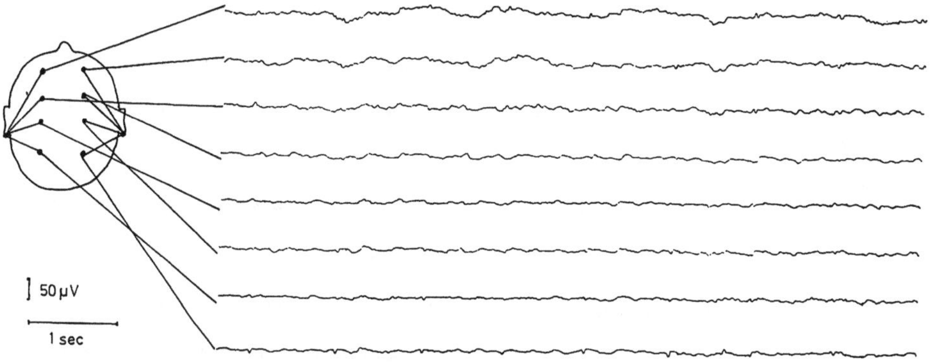

Fig. 3. Low-voltage EEG. Reference (unipolar) leads. Male, 24 years old

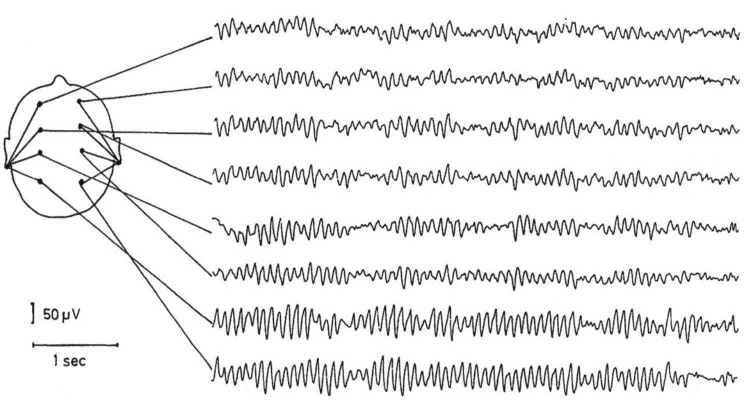

Fig. 4. EEG with monomorphic alpha waves. Reference (unipolar) leads. Male, 22 years old

rying this variant are, on the average, much younger than the population from which they came has suggested that it might disappear during the adult years [8]. This has now been demonstrated by observation of a concordant MZ twin pair, first observed at the age of 15. The variant was seen repeatedly when the twins were in their 20ies but had disappeared almost completely when they were reexamined at the age of 45 [5]. In other instances, however, this variant was shown to have persisted up to a very advanced age.

Two concordant MZ twins were observed. In a few cases, this 4–5 cycle/s variant was found in siblings, and once even in members of two generations of one family [11], Most cases, however, seem to be sporadic [8]. The genetic basis is not yet clear; possibly it is heterogenous. This variant is remarkable because neurovegetative as well as psychological abnormalities, while not always present,

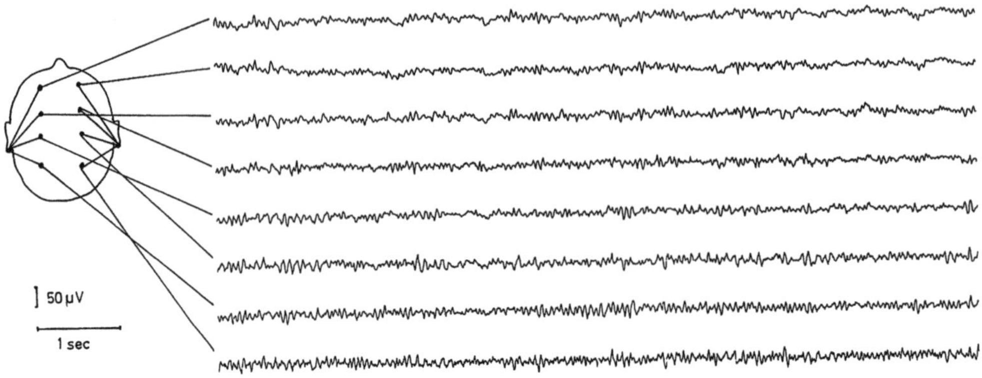

Fig. 5. EEG with 16–19 c/s beta waves (fast alpha variants). Reference (unipolar) leads. Female, 40 years old

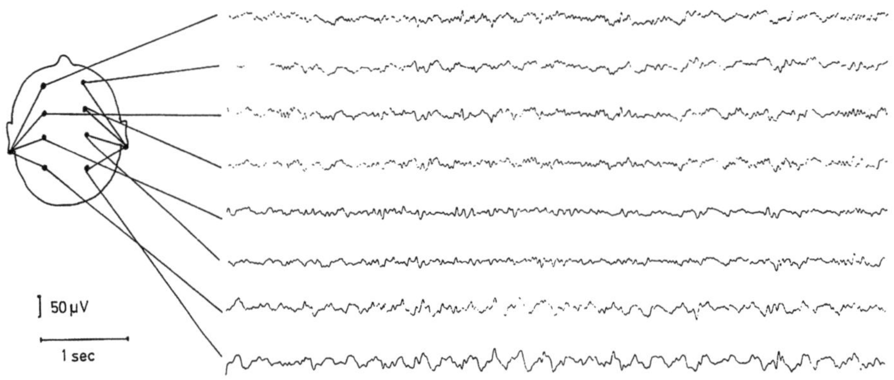

Fig. 6. EEG with 4–5 c/s rhythm. Reference (unipolar) leads. Male, 23 years old

are more common in its carrier than in the general population [10, 25]. In contrast to superficially similar EEG types commonly observed in children with epilepsy (see Doose, this volume), adults showing the 4–5 cycle/s variant appear to have little or no liability to develop epileptic seizures.

The EEG with Beta Waves

While most healthy adults show, in their resting EEG, more or less well-developed alpha activity, a significant admixture of beta waves (>13 cycle/s) is less frequently observed. Even within this group, beta activity shows a high degree of interindividual variation. This variation is influenced strongly by age and sex. EEG records with beta waves become more frequent with advancing age in both sexes, and are generally much more common in females than in males.

Within the heterogenous group of EEGs with beta waves (Fig. 7–9) one type stands out quite clearly. Here, more or less spindle-like groups of (often very fast) beta waves can be seen in frontal and frequently also in precentral leads. This type may be subdivided into two variants. In one of them, beta groups are rare and confined to frontal leads, and beta frequency is very high. In the second variant, the beta groups are much more frequent. Often, they are visible in precentral and sometimes even in central leads. The first of these variants was found in about 0.5%, the second in about 1.5% of normal German males. In both of them, a simple autosomal dominant mode of inheritance was found.

The EEG specialist – especially if he or she is concerned with the diagnosis of epileptics – should be aware of the existence of these variants. Similar but transient beta groups are often seen in subjects treated with antiepileptic or psychotropic drugs. Hence, not every patient who shows beta groups but strongly denies having taken any drugs is a liar. Moreover, we occasionally saw similar beta groups in patients suffering from epileptic fits, even without (known) drug therapy and without additional instances in their families [18].

In most normal subjects with beta waves, however, these waves are mixed more or less diffusely with alpha waves in frontal and precentral leads; they are often more pronounced in occipital leads. There is a continuous range of varia-

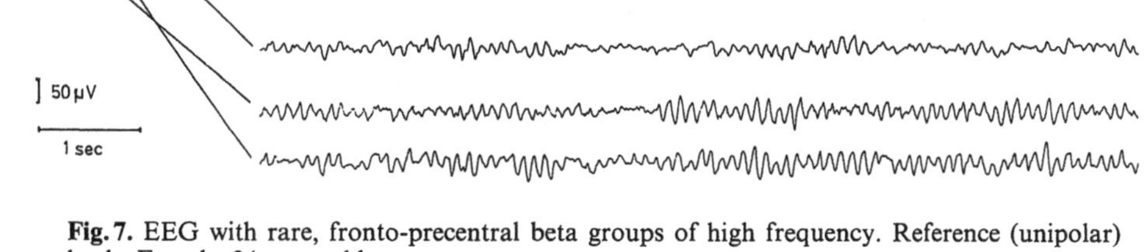

Fig. 7. EEG with rare, fronto-precentral beta groups of high frequency. Reference (unipolar) leads. Female, 24 years old

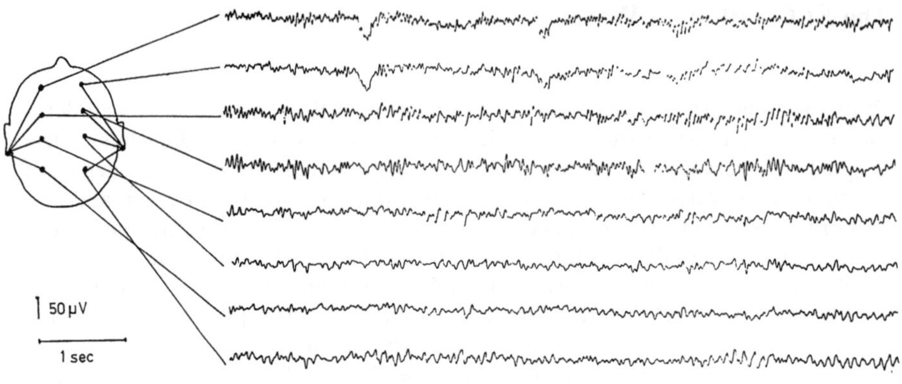

Fig. 8. EEG with numerous, fronto-precentral groups of beta waves. Reference (unipolar) leads. Male, 25 years old

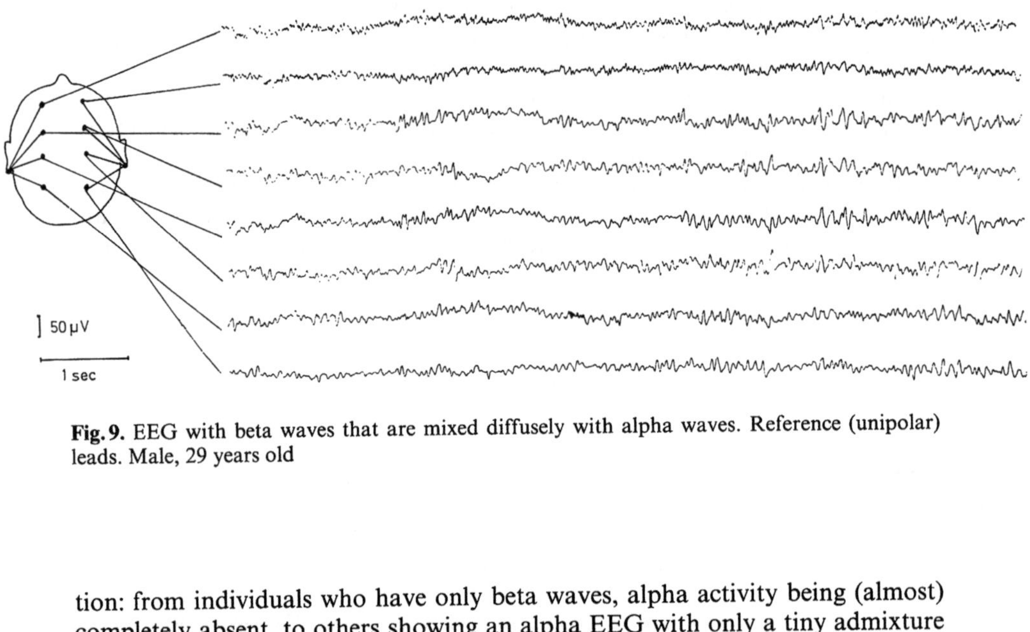

Fig. 9. EEG with beta waves that are mixed diffusely with alpha waves. Reference (unipolar) leads. Male, 29 years old

tion: from individuals who have only beta waves, alpha activity being (almost) completely absent, to others showing an alpha EEG with only a tiny admixture of beta waves, mostly with low amplitudes. This group of EEG records is obviously heterogenous and sometimes not clearly distinguishable from EEG types with no visible beta activity. It is therefore not surprising that the genetic basis is also not clearcut. Prevalence of diffuse beta wave EEGs in first-degree relatives of probands with this EEG type is between twice and three times that of the general population of individuals of the same age and sex: it is highest in mothers, followed by, in order of frequency, daughters, fathers, brothers, and sons [17]. This reflects the above-mentioned observation that the EEG with diffuse beta waves is more common in females than in males and becomes more common with advancing age in both sexes. The results can be explained in a preliminary fashion by assuming multifactorial inheritance in combination with a threshold that is located differently in the two sexes and shifts with advancing age [18], see also [19, 20]. Diffuse beta activity very probably is influenced by the level of tonic arousal in the ascending reticular activating system (ARAS).

There have been very few (if any) studies on genetic variation in the normal EEG outside the EEG variants mentioned above, despite the fact that these variants do not nearly exhaust the actually observed variation. But this variation offers very few if any handles for a more incisive analysis. Correlational studies using parameters such as alpha index, dominant frequencies, amplitudes, and power spectra, as well as application of measures and concepts from biometrical genetics (see, for example [4]) would be possible but would probably not lead to any more specific insights. Therefore, it is not surprising that, so far, nobody has considered it worthwhile to do.

The hereditary EEG variants described above have been used as analytical models of neurophysiological parameters with a clear-cut genetic basis that influences feeling tone, behavior, and performance in humans (for references, see [20, 24]). The EEG has also been used to identify and explain in part an aspect of the genetic susceptibility to alcohol addiction [13, 14]. However, a discussion of these studies in greater detail would go beyond the intentions of this review.

Summary

The interindividual variation of the normal human EEG is caused largely by genetic factors, as shown by extensive studies on monozygotic twins reared together and apart. There are some relatively common hereditary variants of alpha or beta activity in which a simple monogenic mode of inheritance has been demonstrated or is made very likely. No influence of this variation on susceptibility to epileptic seizures has been demonstrated so far.

References

1. Buchsbaum MS (1974) Average evoked response and stimulus intensity in identical and fraternal twins. Physiol Psychol 2:365–370
2. Christian W (1975) Klinische Elektroenzephalographie, 2. Aufl. Thieme, Stuttgart
3. Dustman RE, Beck EC (1965) The visually evoked potential in twins. Electroenceph Clin Neurophysiol 19:570–575
4. Falconer DS (1981) Introduction to quantitative genetics, 2nd edn. Oliver & Boyd, Edinburgh London
5. Heintel H, Schalt E, Vogel F (1986) The 4-5 c/s rhythm – changes in time. Eur Arch Psychiatr Neurol Sci 235:299–300
6. Heuschert D (1963) EEG-Untersuchungen an eineiigen Zwillingen im höheren Lebensalter. Z menschl Vererb Konstitutionslehre 37:128–172
7. Juel-Nielsen N, Harvald B (1958) The electroencephalogram in monovular twins brought up apart. Acta Genet 9:57–64
8. Kuhlo W, Heintel H, Vogel F (1969) The 4-5 c/s rhythm. Electroenceph Clin Neurophysiol 26:613–619
9. Lykken DT, Bouchard TJ (1983/84) Genetische Aspekte menschlicher Individualität. Mannheimer Forum 1983/84:79–117. Boehringer, Mannheim
10. Müller-Küppers M, Vogel F (1965) Über die Persönlichkeitsstruktur von Trägern einer seltenen erblichen EEG-Variante. Jahrbuch Psychol Psychother Med Anthropol 12:75–101
11. Neundörfer B (1970) Über die 4-5 c/s EEG-Grundrhythmusvariante. Nervenarzt 41:321–326
12. Propping P (1977) Genetic control of ethanol action on the central nervous system. Hum Genet 33:309–334
13. Propping P (1984) Genetische Einflüsse bei der Wirkung von Alkohol auf das Gehirn, besonders das EEG, beim Menschen. In: Zang K (ed) Klinische Genetik des Alkoholismus. Kohlhammer, Stuttgart, pp 47–64
14. Propping P, Krüger J, Mark N (1981) Genetic disposition to alcoholism. An EEG study in alcoholics and their relatives. Hum Genet 59:51–59
15. Stassen HH, Lykken DT, Propping P, Bomben G (1988) Genetic determination of the human EEG. Survey of recent results on twins reared together and apart. Hum Genet 80:165–176
16. Vogel F (1958) Über die Erblichkeit des normalen Elektroenzephalogramms. Thieme, Stuttgart
17. Vogel F (1962a) Ergänzende Untersuchungen zur Genetik des menschlichen Niederspannungs-EEG. Dtsch Z Nervenheilk 184:101–111
18. Vogel F (1962b) Untersuchungen zur Genetik der β-Wellen des Menschen. Dtsch Z Nervenheilk 184:137–173
19. Vogel F (1970) The genetic basis of the normal human electroencephalogram (EEG). Humangenetik 10:91–114
20. Vogel F (1986) Grundlagen und Bedeutung genetisch bedingter Variabilität des normalen menschlichen EEG. Z EEG-EMG 17:173–188
21. Vogel F, Fujiya (1969) The incidence of some inherited EEG variants in normal Japanese and German males. Humangenetik 7:28–42
22. Vogel F, Götze W (1959) Familienuntersuchungen zur Genetik des normalen Elektroenzephalogramms. Dtsch Z Nervenheilk 178:668–700
23. Vogel F, Krüger J, Schalt E, Schepank H, Kansteiner V (1980) EEG differences in neurotic as compared with normal twin pairs. Hum Genet 54:327–334
24. Vogel F, Krüger J, Höpp HP, Schalt E, Schnobel R (1986) Visually and auditory evoked EEG potentials in carriers of four hereditary EEG variants. Hum Neurobiol 5:49–58
25. Wolpert E, Neundörfer B, Dompf D, Braun J (1979) Untersuchungen zur Psychopathologie bei Merkmalsträgern der 4-5/s-EEG-Grundrhythmusvariante. Arch Psychiat Nervenkr 226:269–282
26. Zung W, Wilson WP (1967) Sleep and dream patterns in twins: Markow analysis of a genetic trait. Recent Adv Biol Psychiatr 9:119–130

Generalized Spikes and Waves

H. Doose [1] and W. K. Baier [1]

In 1951 – in the early days of clinical electroencephalography – Lennox [21] showed in family and twin studies that the risk for manifesting spikes and waves (SW) is, in part, genetic. In identical twins, he found a concordance rate of 84%, as opposed to 0% in dizygotic twins [22]. Since then, SW have been considered a specific, prototypical marker of the genetic liability to manifest seizures. Familial incidence and distribution of SW are used as one basis for genetic modelling in this context. For the most part, efforts to develop explanatory genetic models have started from the assumption that SW were a genetically simple, homogeneous bioelectric phenomenon. This assumption then led to the concept of a homogeneous *centrencephalic* trait. Later findings, however, disproved this concept: SW during rest and hyperventilation on the one hand and SW elicited by photic stimulation on the other hand could be differentiated genetically [8, 30]. Furthermore, there are a number of arguments supporting the complex and heterogeneous nature of spontaneous – not photically evoked – SW. Meanwhile, this alternative to initial simple assumptions can be supported.

Neurophysiology

Our understanding of the neurophysiological basis of the generation of SW is best represented in the hypotheses of Gloor [15, 16]. He studied the feline generalized penicilline-induced epilepsy, which is, in many aspects, a neurophysiological parallel to human corticoreticular epilepsy. According to Gloor's experiments, cortical spikes occur secondary to thalamocortical volleys in the presence of a diffuse cortical hyperexcitability. These, in turn, activate recurrent inhibitory mechanisms. These concurrent antagonistic events are bioelectrically evident as spikes and waves. Thus Jung and Tönnis' [18] concept of the *Bremswelle* (braking wave) has finally received some of the attention it deserves.

Morphology of the Pattern

The morphology of SW can vary considerably. The 3/s SW complex accompanying classical absences is generally accepted to be its prototype. In absences in early

[1] Abteilung für Neuropädiatrie, Universität Kiel, Schwanenweg 20, D-2300 Kiel.

Genetics of the Epilepsies
Beck-Mannagetta et al. (Eds.)

childhood, the frequency is usually lower than 3/s. In myoclonic absences, there is a series of spikes preceding the wave. In the "awakening epilepsy" with tonic-clonic seizures, the interictal EEG shows very irregular SW patterns. Finally, in early infantile seizures including febrile convulsions, the frequency is higher than 3/s ("theta SW"). Until now it has not been clear whether this variability is significant with respect to genetics.

Incidence

In healthy children aged 1–16 years Gerken and Doose [14] found an average incidence of SW during rest and hyperventilation of 1.8%. The maximum (2.9%) occurred in 7- to 8-year-old children. Eeg-Olofsson et al. [12] reported a slightly higher incidence by including sleep recordings. SW are the principal bioelectric symptom of different types of epilepsies with primarily generalized minor or major seizures. In contrast to epilepsies in the stricter sense, it is impossible to detect SW consistently, sometimes only after repeated EEGs from children with febrile convulsions. In systematic follow-up studies, SW occurred in up to 50% of the cases [5, 9, 13, 19, 20]. For febrile convulsions, the peak age for positive findings occurs around 4 years, in other words, at an age when seizures have already subsided in most patients. SW may occur not only in epilepsies with primarily generalized seizures or in febrile convulsions, but also interictally and in partial epilepsies. But this is, in the individual patient, not consistently the case.

Genetics

The first systematic study of the genetics of SW was presented by Metrakos and Metrakos [24, 25]. The authors included probands suffering from petit mal and/or grand mal seizures, without obvious neuropathology to account for the seizures, and a centrencephalic EEG. In siblings aged 4.5–16.5 years, analogous EEG findings could be detected in up to 40% of the cases, but in older siblings and parents in only 7%. This age dependence was supported by follow-up studies of 94 siblings [26]. The authors concluded that the "centrencephalic trait," not the centrencephalic epilepsy itself, was the expression of an autosomal dominant gene with a distinctly age-dependent penetrance.

The results of Metrakos and Metrakos [25, 26] could not be replicated by other authors, which is certainly due to methodological reasons. Metrakos and Metrakos did, for example, not differentiate between SW during rest or hyperventilation on the one hand, and photically elicited SW on the other. Meanwhile, we know for sure that these patterns are genetically different [8, 30], but this does not explain the whole difference. Therefore, the EEG criteria of Metrakos and Metrakos [24–26] may not be identical to those of other authors in this field.

In Gerken and Dooses' family studies there was a strict differentiation between spontaneous SW (during rest or hyperventilation) and photically induced SW. They found a considerably lower incidence of spontaneous SW and a different age distribution. In 524 siblings of 272 SW-positive probands the maximum

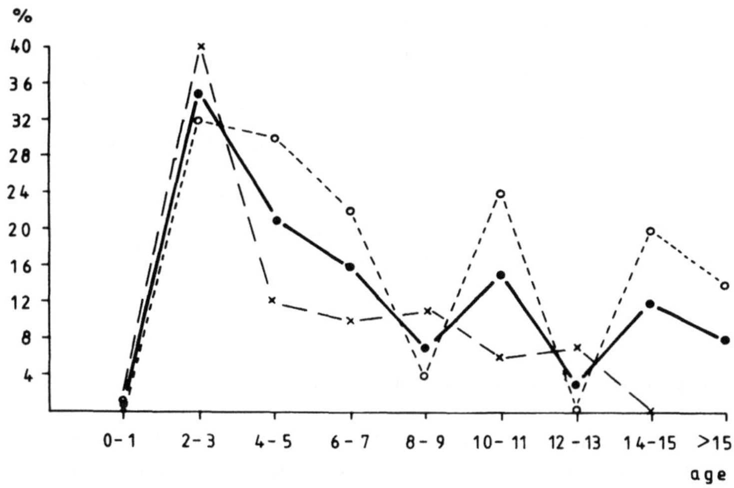

Fig. 1. Frequency of SW in 302 siblings (137 males, 165 females) of probands with primarily generalized minor seizures. ×--× boys; o---o girls; ●——● total

percentage of positive findings was 13%, as opposed to 2.9% in controls. The distribution of the incidence by age was bimodal with a primary peak of 13% between 3 and 6 years of age and a secondary peak of 8% between 13 and 15 years. The lowest frequency was reported for 9- to 10-year-old siblings. In the siblings of female probands the incidence was slightly higher than in the siblings of male probands. Recently, Doose and Baier [10] found similar incidences in 302 siblings of children with primarily generalized minor seizures (Fig. 1). SW are most frequent between 3 and 6 years of age. In 2- to 3-year-old siblings the incidence, maybe due to the small number of probands, is 34%. On the average, only 17% of the 2- to 15-year-old siblings are SW positive. In girls, again, there seems to be a bimodality. Brothers and sisters are affected about equally often. In siblings of female index cases, however, the incidence is higher than in the siblings of male index cases (24% and 11%, respectively; $p < 0.05$). This difference is only due to the sisters of the patients. Tsuboi [32] found a similar relationship to the sex of the index cases in relatives of patients suffering from juvenile myoclonic epilepsy. However, this study did not differentiate between spontaneous and photically induced SW.

Only a few studies of the EEGs from the offspring of SW-positive epileptic patients meet our present standards. For example, Metrakos and Metrakos [25, 26], Tsuboi and Endo [33], and others did not distinguish between photically elicited and spontaneous SW, so their results can hardly be compared with recent findings. Moreover, the pattern's heritability can be estimated only if the index cases are classified exactly. This is fairly easy if the parents suffer from SW epilepsies. However, if the symptomatology is partial, and if the EEG is free of SW in adulthood, no information is provided concerning the state at the age of maximal SW penetrance. So, strictly speaking, the EEG has to be evaluated prospectively, that is, from childhood on in order to meet our standard of parental classification in offspring studies. This is especially restricting in partial epilepsies and in febrile convulsions, once allowance is made for a lower centrencephalic impact in these disorders. For this reason, family findings in epilepsies with partial symptomatology will not be considered in this context [1, 26].

Only the studies of the Heidelberg group yielded representative data for the heritability of spontaneous SW [3, 23, 31]. Children of patients with primarily generalized seizures with spontaneous SW were positive for spontaneous SW in 24% of the cases. The sex of the parent was not significant in this context. These results are roughly equal to the findings of Doose and Baier [10] from siblings of patients with a SW epilepsy.

Heterogeneity of Spikes and Waves

Detailed studies were dedicated to the question of whether SW are a genetically homogenous or heterogenous phenomenon. Rabending and Klepel [30] and Doose and Gerken [8] found support for heterogeneity by demonstrating the independent transmission of photically induced SW and spontaneous SW. Doose and Gerken [8] only included probands if they were unanimously classifiable with respect to the two criteria (Table 1). The findings in siblings were exclusively dependent on the respective pattern in the proband. An interesting parallel emerged from animal experiments: Quesney et al. [27–29] demonstrated that apomorphine, a dopamine receptor agonist, may block photically induced SW in animals as well as in patients while leaving spontaneous SW unaffected.

But there are still other arguments suggesting genetic heterogeneity of SW. Doose et al. [5] found a "peculiar" relationship between SW and a special, genetically determined type of EEG background activity, so-called abnormal theta rhythms (Fig. 2). This rhythmic type of theta background activity is especially typical of epilepsies with primarily generalized seizures in early childhood, but also of febrile convulsions. According to detailed family studies, theta rhythms are the symptom of a – presumably polygenic – disposition to convulsions [6–8]. Theta-positive children with febrile convulsions contract spontaneous SW later on in 63% of the cases. In contrast, only 23% of the children with febrile convulsions, but no theta rhythms, will manifest SW [5]. A different set of 89 children studied recently yielded very similar results (64% and 16%) [9]. Analogous find-

Table 1. Frequency of photoconvulsive reaction in 5- to 6-year-old siblings of probands definitely classified for SW (at rest and hyperventilation) and photoconvulsive reaction (PCR) [8]

Probands EEG	Siblings		
	N	PCR	%
PCR positive/SW positive	163	27	16.6
PCR positive/SW negative	50	11	20.0
PCR negative/SW positive	124	9	7.3
PCR negative/SW negative	49	4	8.2

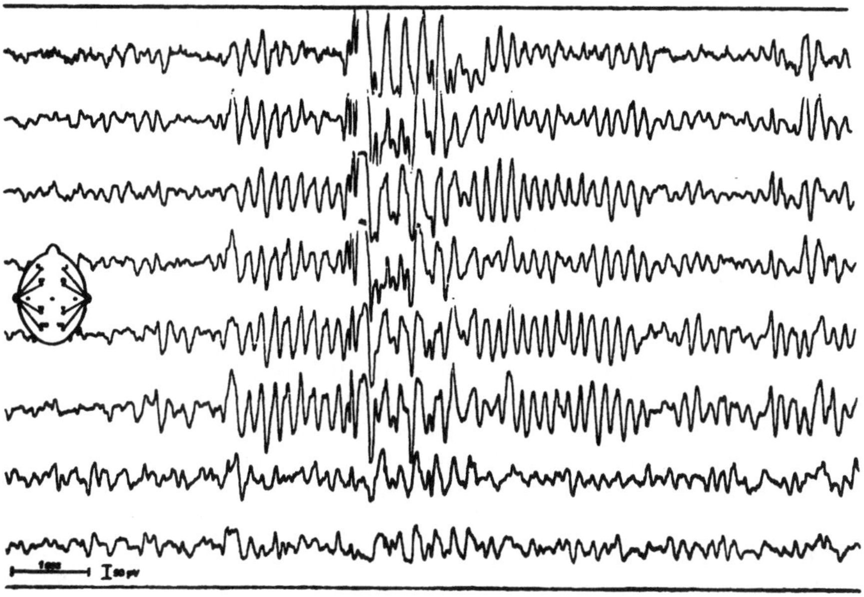

Fig. 2. I.W., male, 10 years old. Myoclonic epilepsy. Bursts of theta with interpolated generalized spikes and waves (time constant 0.1 s)

ings are reported by Doose and Baier [10] in siblings of patients with SW epilepsies with minor seizures. As demonstrated by the statistical analysis of the siblings' EEG data [2], there is a significant association between theta rhythms and spontaneous SW, and, to a lesser degree, also between photically induced SW and spontaneous SW. The most informative finding in this context, however, was the following: Theta rhythms and photically induced SW did not show a statistical interaction. The same genetic independence of photosensitivity and theta rhythms has already been suggested by earlier family studies [8]. Apparently, these phenomena are neither cause-effect related nor just different expressions of one genetic condition. On the other hand, either of these phenomena increases the probability of spontaneous SW. A greater risk, in that sense, is due to theta rhythms than to photically induced SW. The same findings were reported by Gundel and Doose [17], who investigated patients with past febrile convulsions but without epilepsy in the stricter clinical sense.

These results seem to be paradigmatic of the multifactorial background of SW, demonstrating an additive effect of two basic factors. However, one must realize that EEG phenomena like theta rhythms and photically induced SW are not simply expressions of single genetic loci, reducing the complex genetic phenomenon of spontaneous SW to a two-locus anomaly. So in this context, the attribute "basic" is certainly relative. It must be stressed that our method of artificially reducing EEG information to discrete parameters like theta rhythms or even photosensitivity is much too rough biologically. At present, we can only define categories of high and of low expression, which are, for simplicity, designated as "positive" and "negative." In reality, the cut-off point between these categories is certainly pragmatic because it has led to replicable results, but it is arbitrary. Theta rhythms, for example, may "leap to the eye," as in almost all cases of primarily generalized myoclonic-astatic epilepsy, or they may occur in inconspicuous groups, as in many cases of febrile convulsions. Thus, there is good reason to assume that at least the expression of the underlying anomaly is continuous and not just positive or negative.

Much of this may also be true for photosensitivity. Presently, we are studying degrees of expression of this pattern [4] in the relatives of epileptic and nonepileptic photosensitive index cases. Obviously, there are different types of photoresponses, which are determined primarily by the age of the proband, but also reflect the familial liability to convulsions. The high frequency of theta rhythms as well as photosensitivity in healthy children, and the above-mentioned considerations with respect to age dependence and variable expressivity make a polygenic determination of these characters much more plausible than a monogenic trait.

It is an interesting observation that the siblings of patients with primarily generalized seizures in the series studied by Doose and Baier [10] exhibited the qualitatively same EEG phenomena, and that these phenomena were subject to the same pattern of interaction as in patients with febrile convulsions in their later course. This may suggest that the genetic disposition to manifest febrile convulsions is in part identical to the disposition that may give rise to centrencephalic epilepsies in other patients [5, 11, 26]. Moreover, it suggests that the effects of photosensitivity and theta rhythms with respect to SW may represent rather global phenomena, which are not exclusively valid in special nosographic entities. If this view is accepted, it means that we can understand a relatively large amount about the generation of SW, but very little about the large individual variation, reaching from "subclinical" courses in some to literally fatal ones in other patients.

Seizure Risk in Spike-Wave Carriers

For methodological reasons the data presently available are rather imprecise. Most studies did not define the SW pattern exactly, some even dealt only with "epileptiform activity" (for literature, see [31]). Doose and Baier [10] calculated the risk of epileptic seizures in 271 siblings of children suffering from SW epilepsies. A significantly increased risk could only be found in SW-positive siblings (33%), but not in those who were only positive for theta rhythms or photically induced SW (Table 2). Interestingly, the risks were different according to the sex of the index patient (Table 3). The siblings of girls were more often affected than the siblings of boys. This difference holds true even in SW-positive siblings (37% and 25%).

Conclusion. In terms of genetics, spontaneous SW during rest or hyperventilation are not intrinsic phenomena arising "close to gene action." They are nothing more than the expression of a diffuse cortical hyperexcitability in the sense of Gloor [15, 16]. They are obviously not homogeneous. As described above, SW re-

Table 2. EEG findings and seizure risk in 271 siblings of probands with primarily generalized minor seizures [10]

EEG findings	Brothers $N=123$		Sisters $N=148$		Siblings $N=271$	
	N	Seizures (%)	N	Seizures (%)	N	Seizures (%)
Normal	80	5	88	8	168	7
Pathological (total)	43	19	60	17	103	18
SW total	16	38	30	30	46	33
only photo	16	6	24	4	40	5
only theta	11	9	6	0	17	6

Tabelle 3. EEG findings and seizure risk in 271 siblings of male and female probands with primarily generalized seizures [10]

EEG findings	Siblings			
	Of male probands		Of female probands	
	N	Seizures (%)	N	Seizures (%)
Normal	96	5	72	8
Pathological (total)	48	8*	55	26*
SW total	16	25	30	37
Only photo	24	0	16	13
Only theta	8	0	9	11
Total	144	6*	127	16*

* $p<0.05$.

present an epiphenomenon, which arises secondary to a set of mutually independent basic phenomena. These "basic" phenomena are, at least in part, polygenically determined. In trying to formulate an idea about the genetic background of SW, we can conceive a hierarchical structure of sets and subsets of polygenes, the complexity of which is not yet completely understood.

SW are, in conclusion, like the basic characters of theta rhythms and photosensitivity; they are far from specific. Having learned something about their genetic background, we are very much at a loss in trying to explain the extreme variability of the clinical expression of a "SW-type convulsibility" affecting age of onset, clinical symptoms, response to treatment, and so forth.

Summary

This contribution summarizes our present knowledge about the phenomenology, incidence, and, especially, genetics of generalized spikes and waves.

Generalized spikes and waves include genetically heterogeneous phenomena. This is supported by studies demonstrating a largely independent genetic transmission of photically induced spikes and waves (photosensitivity) on the one hand, and spontaneous spikes and waves on the other. In recent studies it has been shown that much of the risk for developing spontaneous spikes and waves is due to a coincidence of photosensitivity and parietal theta rhythms.

In terms of genetics, spontaneous spikes and waves are not intrinsic phenomena arising "close to gene action," but rather represent an epiphenomenon, which arises secondary to a set of mutually independent background liabilities. Earlier hypotheses, assuming an autosomal-dominant, incompletely penetrant centrencephalic trait are not supported by the more recent data.

References

1. Andermann E, Straszak M (1982) Family studies of epileptiform EEG abnormalities and photosensitivity in focal epilepsy. In: Akimoto H, Kazamatsuri H, Seino M, Ward A (eds) Advances in epileptology. XIIIth Epilepsy International Symposium. Raven Press, New York, pp 105–112
2. Baier WK, Doose H (1987) Interdependence of different genetic EEG patterns in siblings of epileptic patients. J Electroenceph Clin Neurophysiol 66:483–488
3. Benninger CK, Matthis P, Scheffner D (1982) EEG findings in children of epileptic parents. In: Anderson VE, Hauser WA, Penry JK, Sing CF (eds) Genetic basis of the epilepsies. Raven Press, New York, pp 95–99
4. Christen H-J, Baier WK, Doose H (1988) Photosensitivity in siblings of photosensitive epileptic and non-epileptic children (in preparation)
5. Doose H, Voelzke E, Petersen CE, Herzberger E (1966) Fieberkrämpfe und Epilepsie. Arch Psychiat Nervenkr 208:400–412, 413–432
6. Doose H, Gerken H, Voelzke E (1968) Genetics of centrencephalic epilepsy in childhood. Epilepsia 9:107–115
7. Doose H, Gerken H, Voelzke E (1972) On the genetics of EEG-anomalies. I. Abnormal theta rhythms. Neuropaediatrie 3:386–401
8. Doose H, Gerken H (1973) On the genetics of EEG-anomalies. IV. Photoconvulsive reaction. Neuropaediatrie 4:162–171
9. Doose H, Ritter K, Voelzke E (1983) EEG longitudinal studies in febrile convulsions. Genetic aspects. Neuropediatrics 14:81–87
10. Doose H, Baier WK (1987) Genetic factors in epilepsies with primarily generalized minor seizures. Neuropediatrics 18 (Suppl I):1–64
11. Doose H, Baier WK (1989) Absences (this volume)
12. Eeg-Olofsson O, Petersen I, Sellden U (1971) The development of the electroencephalogram in normal children from the age of 1 through 15 years. Paroxysmal activity. Neuropaediatrie 2:375–404
13. Frantzen E, Lennox-Buchthal M, Nygaard A (1968) Longitudinal EEG and clinical study of children with febrile convulsions. Electroenceph clin Neurophysiol 24:197–212
14. Gerken H, Doose H (1973) On the genetics of EEG anomalies. III. Spikes and waves in the resting record and/or during hyperventilation. Neuropaediatrie 4:88–97
15. Gloor P (1979) Generalized epilepsy with spike and wave discharge: a reinterpretation of its electrographic and clinical manifestation. Epilepsia 20:571–588
16. Gloor P (1982) Towards a unifying concept of epileptogenesis. In: Akimoto H et al. (eds) Advances in epileptology: XIIIth Epilepsy International Symposium. Raven Press, New York, pp 83–86
17. Gundel A, Doose H (1986) Genetic EEG patterns in febrile convulsions – a multivariate analysis. Neuropediatrics 17:3–6
18. Jung R, Tönnies JF (1950) Hirnelektrische Untersuchungen über Entstehung und Erhaltung von Krampfentladungen: Die Vorgänge am Reizort und die Bremsfähigkeit des Gehirnes. Arch Psychiatr Z Neurol 185:701–735

19. Kajitani T (1984) Different EEG patterns showing the genetic disposition to febrile convulsions. Brain Dev 6:67
20. Laplane R, Salbreux R (1963) Les convulsions hyperpyrétiques. Rev Pract (Paris) 13:753–761
21. Lennox WG (1951) The heredity of epilepsy as told by relatives and twins. J Amer Med Ass 146:529–536
22. Lennox WG (1960) Epilepsy and related disorders. Little, Brown, Boston
23. Lipinsky C, Benninger C, Janz D, Scheffner D, Seminario O, Stolzis L (1976) Historical data and EEG findings in children of epileptic and nonepileptic parents. In: Janz D (ed) Epileptology. Thieme, Stuttgart, pp 29–32
24. Metrakos JD, Metrakos K (1960) Genetics of convulsive disorders. I. Introduction, problems, methods, and base lines. Neurology (Minneap.) 10:228–240
25. Metrakos K, Metrakos JD (1961) Genetics of convulsive disorders. II. Genetic and electroencephalographic studies in centrencephalic epilepsy. Neurology (Minneap.) 11:464–483
26. Metrakos K, Metrakos JD (1974) Genetics of epilepsy. In: Vinken PJ, Bruyn GW (eds) The epilepsies, handbook of clinical neurology, vol 15. North-Holland, Amsterdam, pp 429–439
27. Quesney LF (1984) Pathophysiology of generalized photosensitive epilepsy in the cat. Epilepsia 25:61–69
28. Quesney LF, Andermann F, Lal S, Prelevic S (1980) Transient abolition of generalized photosensitive epileptic discharge in humans by apomorphine, a dopamin-receptor agonist. Neurology 30:1169–1174
29. Quesney LF, Andermann F, Gloor P (1981) Dopaminergic mechanism in generalized photosensitive epilepsy. Neurology 31:1542–1544
30. Rabending G, Klepel H (1970) Fotokonvulsivreaktion und Fotomyoklonus. Altersabhängige genetisch determinierte Varianten der gesteigerten Fotosensibilität. Neuropädiatrie 2:164–172
31. Scheffner D (1982) EEG in offspring (newborns, infants, and children) of epileptic parents. In: Janz D, Bossi L, Dam M, Helge H, Richens A, Schmidt D (eds) Epilepsy, pregnancy and the child. Raven, New York, pp 449–455
32. Tsuboi T (1977) Primary generalized epilepsy with sporadic myoclonias of myoclonic petit mal type. In: Becker PE, Lenz W, Vogel F, Wendt GG (eds) Topics in human genetics, vol IV. Thieme, Stuttgart
33. Tsuboi T, Endo S (1977) Incidence of seizures and EEG anomalies among offspring of epileptic patients. Hum Genet 36:173–189

Photosensitivity

H. Klepel [1] and G. Rabending [2]

Since the introduction of photostimulation as a method of activation into clinical electroencephalography, as well as since the first description of the enhanced electroencephalographic response to light stimuli, i.e., the photoparoxysmal (photoconvulsive) and the photomyogenic (photomyoclonic) reactions, there has been much literature published describing under what conditions these responses are observed, their various manifestations, and in recent years, their clinical relevance.

As proposed by Bickford in 1952 [1], a photoparoxysmal response in the electroencephalogram is defined as the occurrence of generalized, bilaterally symmetrical, regionally pronounced or also focal regular or irregular spike-wave or polyspike-wave complexes in conjunction with light stimulation. It has not yet been elucidated whether or not the various electroencephalographic patterns of the photoparoxysmal response and its varied relationship to the light stimulus (i.e., responses when flickering light stimulation starts, those occurring only after lengthy light stimulation, those that outlast the light stimulus, or those that stop when photostimulation is terminated) have their roots in genetics.

The photomyogenic response is characterized in the electroencephalogram by stimulus-dependent recruiting of rhythmic muscular action potentials. Myoclonias occur either in the light stimulation sequence (i.e., *coup a coup*), or they are triggered by the flashes at a fixed or variable ratio. The photomyogenic response reflects a quantitatively enhanced sensitivity to light. It is the consequence of a disinhibition of the optomotor reflex. Both manifestations may be accompanied by unpleasant and embarrassing subjective sensations and also vegetative sensations such as nausea, sweating, tachycardia, or bradycardia. They are probably due to close relationships between the light stimulation-induced cerebral excitation and the structure of the limbic system, which regulate the vegetative and the circulatory functions.

The photoparoxysmal and the photomyogenic responses occur predominantly in females, which is thought to be for hormonal reasons. Electroencephalographic examinations of the relatives of photosensitive subjects demonstrated that the photoparoxysmal response is a genetically defined electroencephalographic sign with age-dependent and sex-influenced penetrance. Expression occurrs for

[1] Klinik für Neurologie und Psychiatrie, Medizinische Akademie, Leipziger Str. 44, DDR-3090 Magdeburg.
[2] Nervenklinik der Ernst-Moritz-Arndt-Universität, DDR-2300 Greifswald.

Genetics of the Epilepsies
Beck-Mannagetta et al. (Eds.)

the most part in childhood and adolescence. Due to the high incidence in the normal population, the age-dependent penetrance and expressivity, as well as the predominant occurrence in females among photosensitive subjects and their relatives, a polygenetic inheritance is assumed. Electroencephalographic investigations on the genetics of photosensitivity were carried out by many authors, including the following in chronological order: Davidson and Watson (1956) [3], von Hedenström (1968) [8], Doose et al. (1969) [5], (1973) [4] Meldrum (1976) [9], Takahashi (1976) [13], as well as Newmark and Penry (1979) [10].

From our own investigation of 42488 electroencephalograms with photostimulation from 30855 patients, it was determined that the incidence rate of the photoparoxysmal response among probands from all age groups with neurologic-psychiatric disorders was 1.7% [12]. This corresponds to the results of other authors obtained from groups of patients with a comparable line-up and of similar age groups, e.g., 1.6% observed by Buchthal and Lennox [2], 2% by Watson and Davidson [14], and 1.3% noted by Gastaut et al. [6].

The maximum penetrance of the photoparoxysmal response is in the second decade of life, between 10 and 20 years of age. The incidence rates of 6.8% and 2.1% for females and males, respectively, in this age group are in agreement with findings reported in the literature [4, 5, 11, 12].

A statistically significant relationship was found between the photoparoxysmal response and generalized idiopathic epilepsy. Unless epileptic seizures have occurred, the finding of a photoparoxysmal response in the electroencephalogram does not per se justify the diagnosis of epilepsy. But among 513 patients with a photoparoxysmal response (i.e., 1.7% of 30855 patients), an epilepsy was demonstrated in 397 (which is equal to 77.4%), whereas the total number of patients with epilepsy is only 16.9%, that is, 5211 out of 30855 patients [12].

In 1984, Goosses [7, 15] found statistical correlations between photosensitivity, on the one hand, and pyknoleptic absences, awakening grand mal, and juvenile myoclonic epilepsy, on the other hand. The seizure types which are characteristic for these syndromes were also those that are mainly elicited by photostimulation or by ordinary light stimuli.

Although a photoparoxysmal response is tantamount to abnormal photosensitivity, information on the photomyogenic response, its genetic basis, and its relation to epilepsy has remained incomplete. Therefore, a study was performed to determine the relationship of this to patients with a primary generalized predisposition in the electroencephalogram and to investigate the relationships among the photoparoxysmal and the photomyogenic responses.

The incidence of enhanced response to light stimulation in parents, sisters, and brothers of 41 nonphotosensitive patients with a primary generalized predisposition in the electroencephalogram and clinical absences was compared to that in the respective relatives of 101 epileptic patients with photoparoxysmal response [11]. In the control group consisting of relatives of patients with absences, a total of 117 subjects (51 brothers and sisters and 66 parents) were studied electroencephalographically, while in the group of photosensitive subjects the kinship studied by electroencephalography totaled 279 (123 brothers and sisters and 156 parents). The age group range and the sex distribution did not reveal any detectable differences between the groups studied.

Relatives of photosensitive epileptic patients showed a higher rate of photosensitivity than did relatives of nonphotosensitive patients with primary generalized predisposition. This was true for both the incidence of the photoparoxysmal response and the frequency of the photomyogenic response, the former being 15.4% among relatives of photosensitive subjects and the latter being 11.5%. In the control group, however, 4.3% of the relatives studied demonstrated a photoparoxysmal response and 2.6% a photomyogenic response. The differences were statistically significant ($p<0.005$). This suggests that the photoparoxysmal and the photomyogenic responses are genetically independent of the primary generalized predisposition. The average age of relatives with photoparoxysmal response was 20.8 years, while that of relatives with photomyogenic response was 37.4 years.

In the total population of all relatives studied, the relative frequencies of the photoparoxysmal and the photomyogenic responses were found to be inverse in the different age groups. With increasing age the photoparoxysmal response decreased as the photomyogenic response increased. The total mean frequencies of enhanced photosensitivity, determined by summing the relative frequencies of both responses in the individual age groups, do not significantly differ from the mean frequencies of the enhanced photosensitivity for all the relatives. This was checked for age groups that were split both at 10 and 20 years. Hence, it is concluded that both response patterns are age-linked modes of a genetically determined, enhanced photosensitivity. This interpretation is also in accordance with the clinical finding of photogenic tonic-clonic seizures (which also may develop from a photomyogenic response), combinations of both signs which is frequently observed in patients, or a change in manifestation with increasing age.

The greater incidence of photosensitivity in females was confirmed. This sex difference was demonstrated in the brothers and sisters of both groups for the photoparoxysmal response and in the parents for the photomyogenic response which, again, is indicative of the age linkage of both manifestations. Of 313 nonphotosensitive relatives of both groups, 18 (5.8%) had epileptic seizures, whereas 10 (12.1%) of the 83 photosensitive relatives had seizures. This difference was statistically significant ($p<0.025$). Since the incidence of seizures was found to be greater in photosensitive relatives than in nonphotosensitive relatives, it is reasonable to assume that the enhanced photosensitivity is an additional predisposing factor for the clinical manifestation of epileptic seizures.

The photosensitive responses were seen to differ in their biorhythmic behavior. While, in the course of the year, the photoparoxysmal response was noted to be subject to a periodic variation of one cycle per annum, no such periodicity was revealed for the photomyogenic response.

The photomyogenic response is only partially genetically determined; with increasing age, it develops from a photoparoxysmal response. However, the incidence of photomyogenic responses increases in diseases and syndromes with evident brain damage or with impairments of the cerebral cell metabolites. This leads us to the hypothesis that genetically determined photosensitivity differs from that which is mainly induced by brain damage or impairments of the cerebral cell metabolism in its biorhythmic behavior.

This opinion is based on 1035 electroencephalograms with photoparoxysmal response and 1031 electroencephalograms with photomyogenic response, which were recorded within 12 years (mathematical processing was accomplished by distributing over the recording days of the year, POWER spectrum, breaking down the original time series by means of autoregressive analysis, and subsequent filtering).

References

1. Bickford RG, Sam Jacobsen GW, White PT, Daly D (1952) Some observations on the mechanism of photic and photo-Metrazol activation. Electroenceph Clin Neurophysiol 4:275–282
2. Buchthal F, Lennox M (1953) The EEG effect of Metrazol and photic stimulation in 682 normal subjects. Electroenceph Clin Neurophysiol 5:545–558
3. Davidson S, Watson CW (1956) Hereditary light sensitive epilepsy. Neurology (Minneap) 6:235–261
4. Doose H, Gerken H (1973) Fotosensibilität. Genetische Grundlagen und klinische Korrelationen. Z EEG-EMG 4:182–187
5. Doose H, Gerken H, Hien-Völpel KF, Völzke E (1969) Genetics of photosensitive epilepsy. Neuropaediatrie 1:56–73
6. Gastaut H, Trevisan C, Naquet R (1958) Diagnostic value of electroencephalographic abnormalities provoced by intermittent photic stimulation. Electroenceph Clin Neurophysiol 10:194–195
7. Goosses R (1984) Die Beziehung der Fotosensibilität zu den verschiedenen epileptischen Syndromen. Dissertation, Freie Universität Berlin
8. v. Hedenström I (1968) EEG-Befunde bei Sippenangehörigen von Epileptikern. Zbl Neurol Psychiat 7:192
9. Meldrum BS (1976) Experimental epilepsy: its relation to clinical problems. In: Bradford HF, Mardsen CD (eds) Academic Press, London New York San Francisco
10. Newmark ME, Penry JK (1979) Photosensitivity and epilepsy. A review. Raven, New York
11. Rabending G, Klepel H (1970) Photoconvulsive and photomyoclonic reactions: age dependent variations of genetically determined photosensitivity. Neuropaediatrie 2:164–172
12. Rabending G, Klepel H (1978) Die Fotostimulation als Aktivierungsmethode in der Elektroencephalographie. Fischer, Jena
13. Takahashi T, Tsukahara Y (1976) Influence of color on the photoconvulsive response. Electroencephal Clin Neurophysiol 41:113–124
14. Watson C, Davidson S (1957) The patterns of inheritance of cerebral light sensitivity. Electroencephal Clin Neurophysiol 9:378–379
15. Wolf P, Goosses R (1986) Relation of photosensitivity to epileptic syndromes. J Neurol Neurosurg Psychiat 49:1386–1391

Morbidity Risk in Offspring

Genetic Risks in Offspring of Epileptic Parents

T. Tsuboi [1]

Many family studies of epilepsy have been carried out. Alström [1] first investigated 897 families of epileptic probands and found the prevalence of epilepsy in 1.3% of parents, 1.5% of siblings, and 2.9% of offspring; these figures are higher than corresponding figures for the general population. In healthy family relatives of epileptic probands an epileptic EEG abnormality was observed frequently by Metrakos and Metrakos [7].

Previous authors have investigated primarily morbidity risks in the siblings and ancestors of epileptic probands, while few have concerned offspring (Table 1). The present author conducted a pedigree analysis of 2250 epileptic probands at the outpatient clinic of Tsuchida [11], concerning particularly offspring. Genetic risk in offspring is influenced by many factors; these include risk period of morbidity (including or excluding childhood), febrile or neonatal seizures, age at onset of seizures, sex, type of seizures, and pathogenesis (parents) of the probands studied [8]. The present study examines epilepsy (unprovoked nonfebrile recurrent seizures), single nonfebrile seizures, febrile convulsions, and neonatal seizures.

[1] Tokyo Islands Health Center, 3–5–1 Marunouchi, Chiyoda-ku, Tokyo 100, Japan.

Table 1. Incidence of epilepsy among offspring of epileptic probands [11]

Authors	Epilepsy				Febrile convulsions	
	N_1	N_2	n_1	%	n_2	%
Conrad (1940)	1568		70	4.5		
Lennox (1960)	1237		34	2.7		
Annegers et al. (1976)	589		10	1.7	13	2.2
Alström (1950)	825	339	10	2.9		
Harvald (1954)	363	252	12	4.8		
Tsuboi and Christian (1973)	275	103	4	3.9	10[a]	3.6
Tsuboi and Endo (1977)	506	286	12	4.2	34	6.7
Janz and Scheffner (1980)	826	356	26	7.3	27	3.3
Present study	877	545	25	4.6	72	8.2
Median, age-corrected				4.2		3.6

N_1, number of offspring; N_2, number age-corrected after Weinberg's or Strömgren's method; n_1, number with epilepsy; n_2, number with febrile convulsions. [a] Includes childhood convulsions.

Genetics of the Epilepsies
Beck-Mannagetta et al. (Eds.)

Table 2. Incidence of epilepsy and febrile convulsions among sons and daughters of epileptic probands

Offspring	Epileptic fathers ($n=220$)					Epileptic mothers ($n=230$)					Overall	
	N	n_1	%	n_2	%	N	n_1	%	n_2	%	n_1	n_2
Sons	225	6	2.7	19	8.4	213	7	3.3	22	10.3	3.0%	9.4%
Daughters	209	3	1.4	12	5.7	230	9	3.9	19	8.3	2.7%	7.1%
	434	9	2.1	31	7.1	443	16	3.6	41	9.3	2.9%	8.2%

N, total number of offspring; n_1: offspring with epilepsy; n_2, offspring with febrile convulsions.

Results and Discussion

Marriage Rate

The marriage rate of epileptic patients at our outpatient clinic is 53% (257/484) in males and 69% (305/440) in females. Compared with the rates in the general population male patients had a 16% lower rate, but there was no difference in females (69.1% for males, 70.3% for females, age-adjusted). Number of offspring per married patient was 1.6 ± 1.27 (1.7 for male, 1.5 for female), which was lower than that in married brothers and sisters (1.9 ± 1.19, $p < 0.001$). It has been suggested [1, 8–10] that probands' sex and severity of illness influence the risk for offspring. It is assumed that affected men tend to reproduce less than affected women; this, however, is a spurious relationship due to difference in marriage rates between male and female probands.

Epilepsy in Offspring

A total of 450 patients with at least one offspring were selected for the study: 438 sons and 439 daughters (877 total).

The overall incidence of epilepsy was 2.7% for daughters and 3.0% for sons (ns; not statistically significant) – higher in offspring of epileptic mothers than in those of epileptic fathers (3.6% : 2.1%, ns, Table 2). It was highest in daughters of epileptic mothers (3.9%), lower in sons of epileptic mothers (3.3%) and of epileptic fathers (2.7%), and lowest in daughters of epileptic fathers (1.4%).

Febrile Convulsions in Offspring

The overall incidence of febrile convulsions (FC) was 9.4% for sons and 7.1% for daughters (ns). The risk in offspring of epileptic mothers was higher than in those of epileptic fathers (9.3% : 7.1%, ns). It was highest in sons of epileptic mothers (10.3%), lower in sons of epileptic fathers (8.4%) and in daughters of epileptic mothers (8.3%), and lowest in daughters of epileptic fathers (5.7%) (Table 2). The incidence in offspring of parents with a history of FC was higher than in those with no such history (26%, 15/57 versus 7.0%, 57/820; $p < 0.001$). Janz [5] re-

Table 3. EEG abnormality in offspring of epileptic probands. (From Tsuboi [11])

Authors	Type of seizure in probands	Number examined	Epileptic EEG abnormality (%)
Metrakos and Metrakos (1961)	Centrencephalic	82	35.4
Tsuboi and Christian (1973)	Juvenile myoclonic epilepsy	114	24.6
Lipinski (1976)	Absence	71	23.9
	Partial	159	11.3
Grudzinska et al. (1979)		134	39.6
Andermann et al. (1982)	Generalized	82	40.2
	Partial	21	19.0
Tsuboi (1986)	Generalized	128	47.7
	Partial	35	20.0

ported that offspring of parents with a history of FC have a higher incidence of epilepsy than those with no such history (19%, 5/27 versus 3.1%, 18/579; $p<0.001$). This finding, however, was not confirmed in the present study, where the reverse was found to be the case (1.8%, 1/57 versus 2.8%, 24/820; ns). Table 1 presents the age-corrected incidence of epilepsy and FC; the median rate was 4.2% for epilepsy and 3.6% for FC.

Neonatal Seizures in Offspring

Incidence of neonatal seizure in offspring of epileptic probands was 0.12% (1/877); this corresponds to the incidence in the general population (0.13%) in the Fuchu study [11].

Electroencephalography

An epileptic EEG abnormality has frequently been reported in offspring, as shown in Table 3 (only spike and/or spike-and-wave complex was considered as epileptic in this study). The frequency was greater in offspring of probands with generalized epilepsy than in those with partial epilepsy (48% : 20%; $\chi^2=8.646$, $p<0.01$). The rate was higher in offspring of epileptic mothers than in those of epileptic fathers (52% : 27%; $\chi^2=10.815$, $p<0.001$; see Table 4). No difference was found in sons and daughters of epileptic parents (40% : 42%; Table 4). All but one of the 29 families in which at least two offspring were examined showed either epileptic or sharp wave EEG abnormality. These results suggest familial aggregation of EEG abnormalities, as demonstrated by other authors [7, 10]. One may, therefore, presume the existence of families with relatively greater dispositions to epilepsy.

In the present study we found an epileptic EEG abnormality in 7.2% (17/237) of parents, 36% (97/266) of siblings, and 41% (70/171) of offspring of all probands with epilepsy. These frequencies are substantially higher than among controls. Some authors [7, 8] have reported differences in the three generations to depend on the age of subjects: 9.4% in parents, 13.3% in siblings, 24.6% in offspring of probands with juvenile myoclonic epilepsy [9]. A few studies have been conducted on the prevalence of epileptic EEG abnormality in offspring of epileptic probands (Table 3). The prevalence ranged between 11% and 48%, showing a higher figure in the offspring of probands with generalized epilepsy than in those with partial epilepsy [2, 6, 11, and this study].

Incidence of Seizures in Offspring by Type of Seizure in Probands

The incidence of epilepsy in offspring differed by type of seizures in the epileptic probands (Table 4). The risks in offspring of probands with juvenile myoclonic epilepsy, absence, and awakening grand mal were highest (6.7%–15%); such risks in cases with occasional grand mal, diffuse grand mal, and grand mal during sleep were lower (0.7%–5.8%) and in cases with partial epilepsy the lowest (0%–0.6%). The incidence of febrile convulsions was also highest in the first of these groups (7.4%–11%), lower in the second (1.4%–11%), and lowest in the third (3.4%–3.6%). Also the prevalence of epileptic EEG abnormality was highest in the first

Table 4. Incidence of seizures and prevalence of paroxysmal EEG abnormality in offspring of epileptic probands. Each type of seizure was counted if a proband had more than two types

Type of seizure in probands	Sons				Daughters				Offspring					
	N	E	S	EEGp	N	E	S	EEGp	N	E	S	E (%)	FC (%)	EEGp (%)
Awakening GM	99	8	1	13/36	126	7	0	15/30	225	15	1	6.7	10.7	42.4
Absence	14	2	0	5/ 5	16	0	0	2/ 6	30	2	0	6.7	10.0	63.6
Myoclonic PM	17	1	2	6/11	10	3	0	3/ 5	27	4	2	14.8	7.4	56.3
GM	150	1	1	4/10	141	1	1	6/12	291	2	2	0.7	10.4	45.5
GM during sleep	81	0	0	5/16	73	3	0	2/ 9	154	3	0	1.9	2.0	28.0
Diffuse GM	36	1	0	1/ 3	33	3	0	1/ 3	69	4	0	5.8	1.4	33.3
Psychomotor	98	1	3	3/12	77	0	0	2/11	175	1	3	0.6	5.7	21.7
Focal	13	0	0	1/ 2	16	0	0	0/ 4	29	0	0	0	3.6	16.7
	508	14	7	38/95	492	17	1	32/76	1000	31	8	3.1	7.4	40.9
Sex of probands														
Male				12/41 (29.3%)				9/36 (25.0%)						21/77 (27.3%)
Female				26/54 (48.1%)				23/40 (57.5%)						49/94 (52.1%)

N, Number examined; E, with epilepsy; S, with a single nonfebrile seizure; FC, with febrile convulsions; EEGp, epileptic EEG abnormality of spike and/or spike-and-wave complex (positive spikes or small spikes not included).

group (42%–64%), lower in the second (28%–45%), and lowest in the third (17% –22%). These results suggest that regarding genetic aspects there are three categories in epilepsy.

Similar Types of Seizure in Probands and Offspring

Appearance of similar types of epilepsy in family members has been reported. Twenty-five combinations of epileptic probands and offspring in the present study and 26 combinations in Janz's study [5] have been analyzed. Similar types of seizure were observed in all cases in this study, both of primary generalized epilepsy of grand mal seizure in 24 cases and both of partial seizure (focal) in one. Also in Janz's study primary generalized seizure combination was predominantly observed; in offspring of 12 probands with focal seizures, nine with generalized (i.e., dissimilar) seizures, two focal (i.e. similar) seizures, and one unclassified case were found [5].

Age at Onset of Seizure in Probands and Offspring

Age at onset of seizures in probands and in offspring correlated at +0.495 ($p<0.05$) in this study; Janz ascertained a correlation of +0.515 ($n=14$) in the generalized seizure group and +0.463 ($n=12$) in the focal seizure group (calculated by the present author). These figures clearly demonstrate the positive correlation between age at onset of seizures in epileptic probands and that of their offspring. Mean age at onset of epilepsy (excluding FC) was 18.3 ± 11.52 among probands and 10.1 ± 7.78 years among offspring in this study ($p<0.001$). In Janz's study mean ages were 10.6 ± 3.99 and 6.86 ± 4.17 in the generalized seizure group and 22.9 ± 12.07 and 3.8 ± 3.90 years in the focal seizure group (calculated by the present author). There exists a tendency toward anticipation in both groups, as in many genetical diseases, this difference is particularly large in the focal group.

Exogenous Factors

Pre- and perinatal complications were found in 6 of 25 offspring with epilepsy. There was no evidence that perinatal complication increased the risk of epilepsy in the offspring. The incidence of epilepsy is higher ($p<0.001$) in the offspring of probands with unknown exogenous cause (3.3%, 24/727) than in those with known exogenous cause (0%, 0/150).

Genetic Counselling

Incidences of epilepsy, febrile convulsions, and EEG spike abnormality in offspring of epileptic probands with primary generalized epilepsy and awakening grand mal were higher than in those with temporal lobe epilepsy and complex partial seizures (Table 5). In cases of awakening grand mal when both proband and parent had suffered epilepsy, these three rates increased considerably; when proband and one of his siblings had had epilepsy, the risks were rather moderate; and when proband and one second-degree relative had had the illness, the figures were low. In case of complex partial seizure the influence on these rates was only slight as to whether a family member had had epilepsy or not.

Table 5. Incidence of epilepsy, febrile convulsions, and epileptic EEG abnormality among offspring of epileptic probands

Offspring \ Type of seizure in probands		Awakening grand mal				Complex partial seizures			
		Sons	Daughters	Total	Percent	Sons	Daughters	Total	Percent
Number of offspring	(*N*)	99	126	225		98	77	175	
with epilepsy		8	7	15	6.7	1	0	1	0.6
with FC		13	11	24	10.7	8	2	10	5.7
with EEG ab.		13/36	15/30		42.4	3/12	2/11		21.7
Epilepsy in proband and one parent	(*N*)	8	11	19		1	1	2	
with epilepsy		2	3	5	26.3	0	0	0	
with FC		2	1	3	15.8	0	0	0	
with EEG ab.		2/6	3/4		50.0	–	–		–
Epilepsy in proband, neither parent	(*N*)	91	115	206		97	76	173	
with epilepsy		6	4	10	4.9	1	0	1	0.6
with FC		11	10	21	10.2	4	2	6	3.5
with EEG ab.		11/30	12/26		41.1	3/12	2/11		21.7
Epilepsy in proband and one sibling	(*N*)	20	14	34		5	5	10	
with epilepsy		0	1	1	2.9	0	0	0	
with FC		6	0	6	17.6	1	1	2	20.0
with EEG ab.		4/11	1/2		38.5	0/2	0/2		0
Epilepsy in proband and one 2nd-degree relative	(*N*)	7	12	19		4	2	6	
with epilepsy		0	0	0		0	0	0	
with FC		0	1	1	5.3	1	1	2	33.3
with EEG ab.		0/1	1/2		33.3	0/2	–		0

FC, febrile convulsions; EEG ab, epileptic EEG abnormality of the spike and/or spike-and-wave pattern.

Segregation analysis in probands with awakening grand mal showed that the risk was higher when mother had had epilepsy (36%, 5/14) than when father (0%, 0/5) or neither parent had suffered from epilepsy (4.9%, 10/206; $\chi^2 = 19.650$, $p < 0.001$). If one sibling of the probands had had the illness, the risk was 2.9% (1/34). A similar analysis was made on probands with complex partial seizures, and an essentially low risk figures were observed (0.6%, 1/173 and 0%, 0/10, respectively). For genetic counselling these results may be helpful.

Medical Prophylaxis and Genetic Counselling

Medical prophylaxis may effectively reduce the risk that genetic carriers will become manifest. Several factors are known to act as a trigger. As yet, however, we do not have enough knowledge on the basic mechanism in triggering of neurophysiologic condition or neurochemical abnormality clinical manifestation which could lead to preventive measures.

The general risk that an epileptic may have an epileptic offspring is between 1% and 5%. The morbidity risk in the offspring stands at the maximum if both parents (proband and his partner) are epileptic of the primary generalized type, due to unknown exogenous cause, and show spike-wave-complex EEG abnormality. The risk for offspring is least – probably not more than 1% – if the proband had epilepsy of the partial seizure type with known etiology, the marital partner's EEG is normal, and the family history negative.

References

1. Alström CH (1950) A study of epilepsy in its clinical, social and genetic aspects. Acta Psychiat Neurol (suppl) 63:1–284
2. Andermann E, Dansky L, Andermann F, Metrakos JD, Metrakos K (1982) EEG in children of epileptic parents: findings and implications. In: Janz D et al (eds) Epilepsy, pregnancy, and the child. Raven, New York, pp 457–467
3. Annegers JF, Hauser WA, Elveback LR et al. (1976) Seizure disorders in offspring of parents with a history of seizures: a paternal-maternal difference? Epilepsia 17:1–9
4. Grudzinska B, Majchrzak R, Kazibutowska Z (1979) EEG investigations of offspring of epileptic women. Neurol Neurochir Pol 29:625–630
5. Janz D, Scheffner D (1980) Seizures in children of epileptic parents. In: Canger et al. (eds) Advances in epileptology. 11th Epilepsy, international symposium. Raven, New York, pp 311–318
6. Lipinski C, Benninger C, Janz D, Scheffner D, Seminasio O, Stolzis L (1976) Historical data and EEG findings in children of epileptic and nonepileptic parents. In: Janz D (ed) Epilepsy. Thieme, Stuttgart, pp 29–32
7. Metrakos JD, Metrakos K (1961) Genetics of convulsive disorders. II. Genetic and electroencephalographic studies in centrencephalic epilepsy. Neurology (Minneap) 11:474–483
8. Tsuboi T, Christian W (1973) On the genetics of the primary generalized epilepsy with impulsive petit mal type. Humangenetik 19:155–182
9. Tsuboi T (1977) Primary generalized epilepsy with sporadic myoclonias of myoclonic petit mal type. Topics in human genetics IV. Thieme, Stuttgart, pp 1–115
10. Tsuboi T, Endo S (1977) Incidence of seizures and EEG abnormalities among offspring of epileptic parents. Hum Genet 36:173–189
11. Tsuboi T (1986) Seizures of childhood: a population-based and clinic-based study. Acta Neurol Scand 71 (suppl) 110:1–237

Morbidity Risk for Seizures and Epilepsy in Offspring of Patients with Epilepsy

G. Beck-Mannagetta [1], D. Janz [1], U. Hoffmeister [1], I. Behl [1], and G. Scholz [2]

Introduction

For more than a century family studies on the morbidity risk in offspring of patients with epilepsy have contributed to a better understanding of the genetic background of epilepsy and have provided basic data for genetic counseling in this field. The quotations in the review by Newmark and Penry [23] from 1980 date back to 1880, when Eccheverria [15] and Gowers [16] already knew about the increased morbidity in offspring of their epileptic patients. This century has contributed several family studies, mainly on selected populations based on clinic referrals (Table 1) [1, 4, 13, 17, 20, 22, 26]. The more recent studies by Tsuboi and Endo in 1977 [26], Annegers et al. in 1976 [3] and 1978 [4], Janz and Scheffner [20], and Beck-Mannagetta and Lipinski [7] in 1980, and Janz and Beck-Mannagetta [20] and Beck-Mannagetta and Janz [8] in 1982 have confirmed, though based on different populations and referring to different morbidity risk periods, that there is an overall risk of epilepsy in offspring of epileptic parents of between 3% and 4%, and that the risk is even higher for offspring of patients with certain

[1] Neurologische Abteilung, Universitätsklinikum Rudolf Virchow, Freie Universität Berlin, Spandauer Damm 130, D-1000 Berlin 19.
[2] Abteilung für Neurophysiologie, Universitätsklinikum Rudolf Virchow, Freie Universität Berlin, Spandauer Damm 130, D-1000 Berlin 19.

Table 1. Incidence of epilepsy in offspring of epileptic patients

Study	Probands	Offspring		
		Total	Affected	
	N	*N*	*n*	%
Conrad (1937)	519	1568	70	4.5
Alström (1950)	897	239 [a]	10	3.0
Harvald (1951)	162	252 [b]	11	4.4
Lennox (1960)	4231	1237	34	2.7
Tsuboi and Endo (1977)	263	506	12	2.4
Annegers et al. (1978)	336	687	25	3.6
Janz and Scheffner (1980)	384	672	24	3.6

[a] Age corrected by Weinberg's method.
[b] Age corrected by Strömgren's method.

Genetics of the Epilepsies
Beck-Mannagetta et al. (Eds.)

types of seizures. This morbidity risk is 2–4 times greater than that in the general population, based on the assumption that the cumulative incidence of 1.1% by the age of 25 years ascertained from the Rochester population [18] can be used as a comparison for studies performed elsewhere than in the United States.

Though basic data have been available for decades, there remain questions still adequately to be answered using family studies which follow classifications recently defined and accepted systems proposed by the Commission on Classification and Terminology of the International League against Epilepsy [11, 12], and in which heterogeneity is taken into account [2]. The value of the contribution of assessing morbidity risks in offspring of epileptic patients to the study of the genetics of particular seizure types and syndromes is limited not only by the length of follow-up, but also in particular by it being restricted to a selection of those epileptic patients who are able to reproduce. The proportion of patients with epilepsy of early onset is necessarily low in a population of patients that can reproduce, on one hand because some syndromes like Rolandic epilepsy have a favorable prognosis and the patients do not need medical care at reproductive age, and on the other hand because the severity of other syndromes like West and Lennox-Gastaut syndrome and their effects on social behavior hinder the patients, especially men, in marrying and having children [14]. The latter effect may contribute to the maternal preponderance in the transmission of epilepsy [24].

Material and Methods

This study on risks to offspring is an update of previously published data, with the advantage that there has been a follow-up period of 20 years in more than 50% of the cases and of at least 15 years in 80%. The study should contribute to empirical prognosis for subclinical (see Tsai et al., this volume) and clinical signs and symptoms of epilepsy, and is based on an investigation of 434 families with parents affected by epilepsy (in the sense of having had at least two unprovoked epileptic seizures) and the 858 offspring. Probands were enrolled from 1969 to 1972 and from 1979 to 1982 in the outpatient clinics for epilepsy at the Universities of Heidelberg and Berlin by asking random patients with children under 16 years of age if they and their children would join the study. Families in which both parents were affected were considered, although this is not proven, a special problem and were excluded from the analysis. The remaining 840 children from 427 families were followed up regularly once a year or once every two years, and at least twice during the follow-up period. On each occasion the seizure diagnosis of the affected parent was updated, and the child's development including seizures, physical condition, and EEG was noted. The data were recorded in a standardized form compatible for computer analysis by SPSS [10]. Selected frequency tables were compared by chi-square test [25].

Results

Overall 9.3% of the offspring suffered seizures, i.e., 90.7% remained healthy in this respect during the follow-up period (Fig. 1).

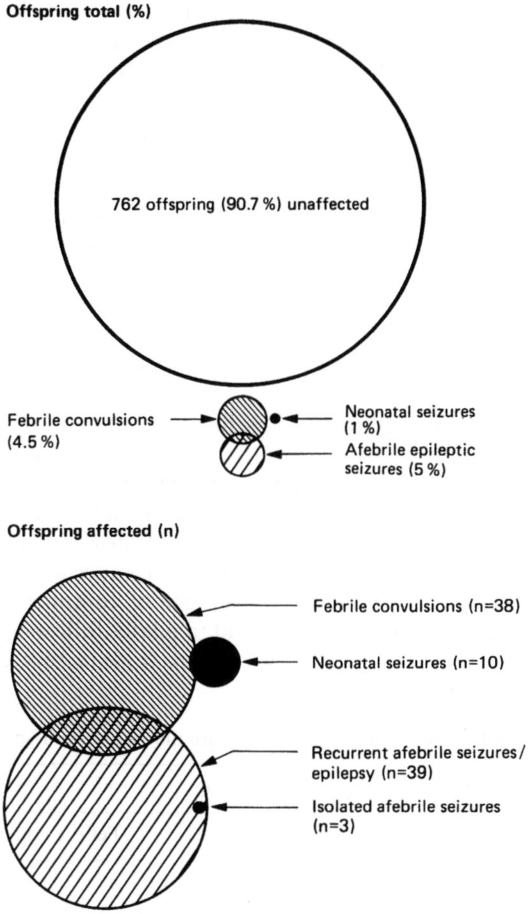

Fig. 1. Morbidity risk in offspring of epileptic parents

There were 10 cases of *neonatal seizures,* i.e., 1.2%, which is in the normal range found in the general population [28].

Febrile convulsions occurred in 38 children, i.e., 4.5%, which lies within the upper part of the range of figures for North American and Western European populations [19]. These 38 cases were split up into two groups because of differences in the prognostic implications. Twenty-eight of the children experienced febrile convulsions alone (3.3%), but in the other 10 cases the febrile convulsions were followed by recurrent afebrile epileptic seizures (1.2%). These 10 cases comprised a quarter of the total number of cases of epilepsy in the offspring. Ten out of 38 patients with febrile convulsions developing unprovoked afebrile seizures is a considerably higher proportion than is found in epidemiological studies, where epilepsy is found to follow febrile convulsions in 2%–4.4% [5, 27]. According to a recent follow-up till the age of 25, 7% of patients who have febrile convulsions develop unprovoked seizures [6], but among these, those with complex features to their febrile convulsions have a higher risk of unprovoked seizures (17%–22%). This figure is close to that for the offspring of epileptic parents affected by febrile convulsions followed by epilepsy, but the unfavorable prognosis of febrile convulsions in these cases cannot be explained solely by a high proportion having fits with complex features.

The overall risk of *afebrile seizures* (5%; 42/840) approaches the risk figures given in early retrospective studies on adult offspring of patients with epilepsy [23]. Disregarding isolated seizures ($n=3$), the remaining risk for *epilepsy*, in the sense of recurrent unprovoked seizures, whether preceded by febrile convulsions or not, is 4.6% (39/840). Compared to the results of the previous updates of the same study [20, 21], the relative risk is, as expected, increasing with duration of follow-up.

After assessing the baseline risk, two major questions arise: (1) Are there special factors – parent or offspring related – that contribute to the risk and (2) Are there factors which enable predictions to be made about the types of seizures in the offspring, including their course and prognosis.

The search for special factors follows, as in previous such attempts [9], the classic dichotomies of presence or absence of seizures or seizure syndromes in the parents, and presence or absence of complications during pregnancy, delivery, and the neonatal period, and in a later follow-up period, in the offspring. Correlations were searched for between these factors and outcome in terms of presence

Table 2. Sex of proband and seizure morbidity in offspring

Sex of proband	Offspring				
		Febrile convulsions[a]		Epilepsy[b]	
	N	*n*	%	*n*	%
Male	387	15	3.9	13	3.4
Female	453	23	5.1	26	5.7

[a] Febrile convulsions including febrile convulsions followed by afebrile seizures.
[b] Epilepsy including febrile convulsions followed by afebrile seizures.

Table 3. Etiology of parents' epilepsy and seizure morbidity in offspring

Etiology in parents' epilepsy	Offspring				
		Febrile convulsions[a]		Epilepsy[b]	
	N	*n*	%	*n*	%
Known	95	3	3.2	2	2.1
Unknown	745	35	4.7	37	5.0

[a, b] See Table 2.

or absence of febrile convulsions and/or epilepsy; those children with epilepsy following febrile convulsions were included in both groups.

Differentiation by sex of the affected parent confirmed that there is a higher risk of febrile convulsions and/or epilepsy in offspring of women with epilepsy than in offspring of men with epilepsy (Table 2).

Parental epilepsy of unknown etiology is associated with a higher risk of seizures in offspring than parental epilepsy of known etiology (Table 3). The risk is higher for offspring of patients with generalized epilepsy (Table 4). A so far unexplained high risk of seizures was found in the offspring of the small group of patients with epilepsy with generalized and focal features.

Different seizure types have different genetic impacts with respect to morbidity risk in offspring. Concerning febrile convulsions, the highest risk is associated with absence seizures in the parents and the lowest with parental complex focal seizures. For epilepsy, the highest risk is again in offspring of parents with absence seizures and the lowest is associated with parents who have simple focal seizures, whether or not these evolve into generalized tonic-clonic seizures (Table 5). An

Table 4. Type of epilepsy in the parents and seizure morbidity in offspring

Type of epilepsy in parents	Offspring				
		Febrile convulsions[a]		Epilepsy[b]	
	N	*n*	%	*n*	%
Generalized	465	28	6.0*	22	4.7
Focal	361	10	2.8*	14	3.9
Generalized + focal	14	0	–	3	21.4

* $p<0.05$.
[a, b] See Table 2.

Table 5. Parent's seizure type and seizure morbidity in offspring

Seizure type in parents	Offspring				
		Febrile convulsions[a]		Epilepsy[b]	
	N	*n*	%	*n*	%
Generalized					
GTC on awakening and GTC < 7	112	8	7.1	6	5.4
Absences total	177	13	7.3	10	5.7
Absences (childhood) ± GTC	103	6	5.8	7	6.8
Absences (juvenile) ± GTC	74	7	9.5*	3	4.2
JME ± GTC ± absences	110	3	2.7*	3	2.7
Focal					
Simple focal ± focal GTC	91	5	5.4*	2	2.2
Complex focal ± focal GTC	270	5	1.9*	10	3.7

* $p<0.05$.
[a, b] See Table 2.

Table 6. Age of parents at onset of epilepsy and seizure morbidity in offspring

Age at onset in parents (years)	Offspring				
		Febrile convulsions[a]		Epilepsy[b]	
	N	n	%	n	%
0–19	540	30	5.6*	29	4.8
20–	300	8	2.7*	10	3.3

* $p<0.05$.
[a, b] See Table 2.

Table 7. Parental history of febrile convulsions and seizure morbidity in offspring

Febrile convulsions in parents	Offspring				
		Febrile convulsions[a]		Epilepsy[b]	
	N	n	%	n	%
Yes	47	7	14.9*	3	6.4
No	793	31	3.9*	36	4.5

* $p<0.05$.
[a, b] See Table 2.

overrepresentation of female probands in the group of patients with absence seizures (29% male versus 71% female, compared to 41% male versus 59% female in the total study population) may contribute considerably to the apparent higher risk of epilepsy in offspring of women with epilepsy than in offspring of men with epilepsy (see above).

As was found in earlier studies, age of onset of epilepsy in the parent correlates with the morbidity risk in the offspring, there being a significantly lower risk of febrile convulsions as well as of epilepsy for offspring of parents with late onset epilepsy (Table 6). Parental history of febrile convulsions is significantly associated with a higher rate of febrile convulsions in the offspring but shows no obvious relation to the risk of epilepsy (Table 7).

The influence of factors used as indirect measures of the severity of the illness like generalized tonic-clonic seizures occurring during pregnancy and the taking of antiepileptic drugs in pregnancy by epileptic women remains unclear. The only remarkable difference found is that there is a higher risk of febrile convulsions when the mother has taken antiepileptic drugs during pregnancy.

In addition to parental factors, offspring-related factors are also correlated with the morbidity risk. There is no difference attributed to sex of the offspring, but the occurrence of pre-, peri-, and postnatal complications favors the manifestation of epilepsy, although not that of febrile convulsions (Table 8).

Assessment of risk figures and associations between conditions is not all that must be considered. Whether a risk is tolerable or even negligable cannot be mea-

Table 8. Pre-, peri-, and postnatal complications and seizure morbidity in offspring

Risks	Offspring				
		Febrile convulsions[a]		Epilepsy[b]	
	N	*n*	%	*n*	%
Yes	173	11	6.4	14	8.1*
No	667	27	4.1	25	3.7*

* $p<0.05$.
[a,b] See Table 2.

sured exclusively by the size of the risk, because related factors such as social disabilities may be of more importance to the families than the relative risk itself. A certain relationship between age of onset in parents and in affected offspring is common in hereditary diseases and is called anticipation. This was seen with only three exceptions in this study. Onset of disease occurred at only a slightly earlier age than in the parents in offspring of parents with generalized seizures, while onset of seizure disorders in offspring of parents with focal seizures tended to start earlier, up to 20 years or more earlier than the onset of epilepsy had been in the parent. Concerning seizure type in parents and offspring, a homophenous pattern of transmission seems to prevail. Generalized seizures in parents tend to be associated with generalized seizures in offspring. In most cases there are even identical seizure types, although modifications are possible, in this study mainly restricted to children with a history of febrile convulsions. Even in the group of parents with focal epilepsy there is a tendency to homophenous transmission, complex partial seizures being transmitted in this way in three families.

Conclusions

In this study the morbidity risk in offspring of people with epilepsy has been assessed over a reasonably long follow-up and using recent definitions of disease. The study is supplemented by an investigation of subclinical signs (see Tsai et al., this volume) and by a strictly prospective study, the results of which are part of the collaborative study by Granström et al. (this volume). These studies provide useful clues for genetic counseling and the information obtained may also be helpful in designing other genetic studies on special syndromes.

References

1. Alström CE (1950) A study of epilepsy in its clinical, social and genetic aspects. Acta Psychiatr Neurol [suppl] 63:1–284
2. Anderson VE (1982) Family studies of epilepsies. In: Anderson VE, Hauser WA, Penry JK, Sing CF (eds) Genetic basis of the epilepsies. Raven, New York, pp 103–112

3. Annegers JF, Hauser WA, Elveback LR, Anderson VE, Kurland LT (1976) Seizure disorders in offspring of parents with a history of seizures – a maternal-paternal difference? Epilepsia 17:1–9
4. Annegers JF, Hauser WA, Elveback LR, Anderson VE, Kurland LT (1978) Congenital malformations and seizure disorders in the offspring of parents with epilepsy. Int J Epidemiol 7:241–247
5. Annegers JF, Hauser WA, Elveback LR, Kurland LT (1979) The risk of epilepsy following febrile convulsions. Neurology 29:297–303
6. Annegers JF, Hauser W, Shirts SB, Kurland LT (1987) Factors prognostic of unprovoked seizures after febrile convulsions. N Engl J Med 316:493–498
7. Beck-Mannagetta G, Lipinski C (1980) Febrile convulsions among children of parents with epilepsy. In: Canger R, Angeleri F, Penry JK (eds) XIth epilepsy international symposium. Raven, New York, pp 367–369
8. Beck-Mannagetta G, Janz D (1982) Febrile convulsions in offspring of epileptic probands. In: Anderson E, Hauser WA, Penry JK, Sing CF (eds) Genetic basis of the epilepsies. Raven, New York, pp 145–150
9. Beck-Mannagetta G, Janz D (1985) Bedingungen für die Manifestation einer genetischen Anfallsbereitschaft. In: Hallen O, Meyer-Wahl JG, Braun J (eds) Epilepsie 83. Einhorn, Reinbek, pp 32–39
10. Beutel P, Schubö W (1983) SPSS-9, Statistik-Programm-System für die Sozialwissenschaften. Fischer, Stuttgart
11. Commission on Classification and Terminology of the International League against Epilepsy (1981) Proposal for revised clinical and electroencephalographic classification of epileptic seizures. Epilepsia 22:489–501
12. Commission on Classification and Terminology of the International League against Epilepsy (1985) Proposal for classification of epilepsies and epileptic syndromes. Epilepsia 26:268–278
13. Conrad K (1937) Erbanlage und Epilepsie. IV. Ergebnisse der Nachkommenschaftsuntersuchungen an Epileptikern. Z Ges Neurol Psychiatr 155:521–581
14. Dansky LV, Andermann E, Andermann F (1980) Marriage and fertility in epileptic patients. Epilepsia 21:261–271
15. Eccheverria MG (1980) Marriage and hereditariness of epileptics. J Med Sci 26:346–369
16. Gowers WR (1881) Epilepsy and other chronic convulsive diseases. Wood, New York
17. Harvald B (1951) On the genetic prognosis of epilepsy. Acta Psychiatr Scand 26:339–352
18. Hauser WA, Kurland LF (1975) The epidemiology of epilepsy in Rochester, Minnesota, 1935 through 1967. Epilepsia 21:399–412
19. Hauser WA (1981) The natural history of febrile seizures. In: Nelson KB, Ellenberg JH (eds) Febrile seizures. Raven, New York, pp 5–17
20. Janz D, Scheffner D (1980) Seizures in children of epileptic parents. In: Canger B, Angeleri F, Penry JK (eds) XIth epilepsy international symposium. Raven, New York, pp 311–318
21. Janz D, Beck-Mannagetta G (1982) Epilepsy and neonatal seizures in the offspring of parents with epilepsy. In: Anderson E, Hauser WA, Penry JK, Sing CF (eds) Genetic basis of the epilepsies. Raven, New York, pp 135–143
22. Lennox WG (1960) Epilepsy and related disorders, vol 2. Little, Brown, Boston
23. Newmark ME, Penry JK (1980) Genetics of epilepsy: a review. Raven, New York
24. Ottman R, Hauser WA, Susser M (1985) Genetic and maternal influences on susceptibility to seizures. Am J Epidemiol 122:923–939
25. Sachs L (1984) Angewandte Statistik. Springer, Berlin Heidelberg New York
26. Tsuboi T, Endo S (1977b) Incidence of seizures and EEG abnormalities among offspring of epileptic patients. Hum Genet 36:173–189
27. Tsuboi T, Yamamura K (1978) Febrile convulsions followed by nonfebrile convulsions: analysis based on a maximum likelihood method and discriminant function. Neuropädiatrie 9:103–108
28. Woodbury LA (1978) Incidence and prevalence of seizure disorders including the epilepsies in the United States of America. In: US Department of Health, Education and Welfare (ed) Plan for nationwide action on epilepsy, vol 4. DHEW Publication no. 78–279, pp 24–77

Generalized Spike and Wave Paroxysm – Subclinical Signs of Seizure Liability in Offspring of Epileptic Patients

J. J. TSAI [1], G. BECK-MANNAGETTA [2], D. JANZ [2], D. SCHEFFNER [3], I. BEHL [2], and G. SCHOLZ [4]

Knowledge of the genetics of special electroencephalographic (EEG) patterns related to epilepsy was in the past three decades obtained from family studies of siblings of probands with epilepsy. Bilaterally synchronous generalized spike and wave (GSW) paroxysms during rest and hyperventilation [9, 12], photosensitivity [10], 4–7 rhythms [8], and focal sharp waves [5, 6] have been found to be genetically determined. Suggestions about the mode of transmission of these EEG patterns have also been made. Subsequently, family EEG investigations have focused on children of epileptic patients. Scheffner [20] has critically reviewed these investigations and highlighted some important directions for further study. Although the frequency of specific EEG abnormalities has been reported in these studies, a systematic evaluation of GSW paroxysm has never been carried out. Furthermore, the clinical significance of GSW paroxysms in offspring of epileptic patients has also not been elucidated.

The aims of this study were to determine and characterize the clinical parameters affecting the occurrence of GSW paroxysms and to analyze the natural course of the finding, as well as to evaluate the clinical significance of GSW paroxysms in children of epileptic patients.

Material and Methods

Preliminary EEG findings of the collaborative family study in Heidelberg and Berlin have been reported elsewhere [3, 4, 15]. In this study, all the original EEGs are reevaluated with special attention to GSW paroxysm that occurs only in a waking state and with hyperventilation. Bilaterally synchronous GSW at 2.5–3.5/s, slow SW, fast SW, and polyspike waves without evidence of focal onset are considered GSW paroxysms. Incomplete generalization of SW is not included. 1024 EEGs from 414 children of 95 fathers and 155 mothers from 250 families

[1] Department of Neurology, College of Medicine, National Cheng Kung University, Tainan, Taiwan 70101, R.O.C.
[2] Neurologische Abteilung, Universitätsklinikum Rudolf Virchow, Freie Universität Berlin, Spandauer Damm 130, D-1000 Berlin 19.
[3] Neuropädiatrische Abteilung, Universitätsklinikum Rudolf Virchow, Freie Universität Berlin, Spandauer Damm 130, D-1000 Berlin 19.
[4] Abteilung für Neurophysiologie, Universitätsklinikum Rudolf Virchow, Freie Universität Berlin, Spandauer Damm 130, D-1000 Berlin 19.

Genetics of the Epilepsies
Beck-Mannagetta et al. (Eds.)

Table 1. Number of EEG examinations in the offspring of parents with epilepsy

Number of EEGs	Sons of male patients $n=73$	Daughters of male patients $n=94$	Sons of female patients $n=132$	Daughters of female patients $n=115$	Total $n=414$
One	46 (63.0%)	50 (53.2%)	64 (48.5%)	62 (53.9%)	222 (53.6%)
Two	10 (13.7%)	11 (11.7%)	19 (14.4%)	17 (14.8%)	57 (13.8%)
Three	4 (5.5%)	6 (6.4%)	12 (9.1%)	5 (4.3%)	27 (6.5%)
Four and more	13 (17.8%)	27 (28.7%)	37 (28.0%)	31 (27.0%)	108 (26.1%)

Table 2. Age distribution at the time of each EEG examination

Age (years)	Sons of male patients	Daughters of male patients	Sons of female patients	Daughters of female patients	Total
0–4	26 (16.3%)	52 (20.9%)	132 (40.1%)	124 (43.4%)	334 (32.6%)
5–9	56 (35.0%)	72 (28.9%)	101 (30.7%)	92 (32.2%)	321 (31.3%)
10–14	52 (32.5%)	70 (28.1%)	65 (19.8%)	52 (18.2%)	239 (23.3%)
15–19	25 (15.6%)	45 (18.1%)	28 (8.5%)	17 (5.9%)	115 (11.2%)
≧20	1 (0.6%)	10 (4.0%)	3 (0.9%)	1 (0.3%)	15 (1.5%)
Total	160 (15.6%)	249 (24.3%)	329 (32.1%)	286 (27.9%)	1024 (100.0%)

with one epileptic parent were available for the study. The descendants received at least one EEG examination and a few were regularly examined after birth at the ages of about 6 months, 1 year, 2 years, and so on. The number of EEG examinations is shown in Table 1. Of the offspring, 53.6% had only one EEG and 26.1% had at least four EEGs. The average number of EEGs for each offspring was 2.5. The EEGs were carried out in offspring aged between 6 months and about 20 years. The age distributions at the time of each EEG examination are listed in Table 2. Around two-thirds of the EEGs were performed between 6 months and 9 years of age. EEGs of offspring of women with epilepsy were carried out more frequently in this age range and consequently the group is underrepresented between 10 and 19 years of age.

Each parent had had at least two epileptic seizures. Of the 250 parents 142 (56.8%) had generalized epilepsy. 52 (20.8%) had had generalized tonic clonic seizures (GTCS) only. Pyknoleptic absence (childhood absence) epilepsy was diagnosed in 32 (12.8%) parents, nonpyknoleptic absence (juvenile absence) epilepsy in 29 (11.6%), and impulsive petit mal (juvenile myoclonic) epilepsy in 25 (10.0%). The last three seizure types were mostly combined with grand mal. Focal epilepsy was found in 99 (39.6%) parents, mostly with complex focal seizures, and 9 (3.6%) parents had forms of epilepsy with both generalized and focal seizures (Table 3). The discrepancy in numbers compared to the clinical findings reported by Beck-Mannagetta et al. (this volume) is due to the fact that fewer EEG recordings were available than clinical evaluations.

Table 3. Type of epilepsy in parents

Type of epilepsy	Father $n=95$	Mother $n=155$	Total $n=250$
Epilepsy with generalized seizures	50 (52.6%)	92 (59.4%)	142 (56.8%)
West and Lennox syndrome	3 (3.2%)	1 (0.6%)	4 (1.6%)
Pyknoleptic absences	9 (9.5%)	23 (14.8%)	32 (12.8%)
Nonpyknoleptic absences	8 (8.4%)	21 (13.5%)	29 (11.6%)
Impulsive petit mal	12 (12.6%)	13 (8.4%)	25 (10.0%)
GTCS	18 (18.9%)	34 (21.9%)	52 (20.8%)
Epilepsy with focal seizures	43 (45.3%)	56 (36.1%)	99 (39.6%)
Simple focal seizures	7 (7.4%)	15 (9.7%)	22 (8.8%)
Complex focal seizures	36 (37.9%)	41 (26.5%)	77 (30.8%)
Epilepsy with generalized and focal seizures	2 (2.1%)	7 (4.5%)	9 (3.6%)

Table 4. Frequency of generalized spike and wave paroxysm in the offspring of parents with epilepsy

Parent	Offspring		
	Sons	Daughters	Total
Father	4/ 73 (5.5%)	7/ 94 (7.4%)	11/167 (6.6%)
Mother	7/132 (5.3%)	13/115 (11.3%)	20/247 (8.1%)
Total	11/205 (5.4%)	20/209 (9.6%)	31/414 (7.5%)

Frequency of GSW Paroxysm

The data on GSW paroxysms refer to the first documentation of GSW paroxysm in the EEG examination(s). We avoid using the term of incidence, which is inappropriate in this kind of study. Of 414 descendants of one epileptic parent, 7.5% had GSW paroxysms in at least one EEG (Table 4). Although no parallel control group is available for comparison, there are a few EEG studies of normal children and juveniles with different age ranges. The frequency of GSW paroxysms ranges from 0.3% to 1.8% according to these studies [7, 11, 12, 15, 27]. These figures are actually lower than those found here. However, there are no directly comparable data on the frequency of GSW paroxysms among offspring of epileptic patients. Wide variation in the frequency of GSW paroxysm has been found in a few large series (Table 5), and there are many possible causes of this.

Criteria of GSW Paroxysm

We have defined GSW paroxysm strictly as paroxysm that appears in the EEG examination only at rest and during hyperventilation. GSW paroxysm provoked

Table 5. Frequency of specific EEG abnormalities among offspring of epileptic probands

Research center and reference	Probands		Offspring		
	Type of epilepsy	No.	Total	With specific EEG abnormality	
				n	%
Tokyo					
Tsuboi et al. [26]	Generalized	63	102	38	37.3[a]
Tsuboi [24]	Generalized		128	61	47.7[a]
	Focal		35	7	20.0[a]
Montreal					
Metrakos et al. [18]	Centrencephalic	38	82	29	35.4[b]
Andermann et al. [1]	Focal	60	21	2	9.5[b]
Heidelberg-Berlin					
Lipinski et al. [15]	Epilepsy		275	40	14.5[c]
Benninger et al. [4]	Epilepsy		500	90	18.0[c]
Tsai et al. (present study)	Epilepsy	250	414	31	7.5[d]

[a] Generalized and focal specific abnormality.
[b] Centrencephalic EEG.
[c] Generalized spike and wave, including diffuse spikes and sharp waves.
[d] Generalized spike and wave, excluding diffuse spikes and sharp waves.

by photic stimulation alone is excluded because it differs genetically from that which appears at rest and during hyperventilation [10, 19]. Metrakos and Metrakos [17, 18] made no distinction between them. It is well known that GSW activity can be provoked in a drowsy state and during sleep. However, this kind of provocation does not reflect the biological circadian modulation of GSW activity [14].

Regarding specific EEG abnormalities, Tsuboi [22–25], included bursts with spike(s) of generalized and focal origin in his definition of GSW paroxysm. Both the inclusion of sleep records and the broad definition of the specific EEG abnormalities could be responsible for the surprisingly high frequency of GSW paroxysms in his reports. GSW paroxysms in previous reports from the collaborative study in Heidelberg and Berlin included regular and irregular SW paroxysm as well as diffuse spikes and sharp waves [3, 4, 15]. We have now excluded diffuse spikes and sharp waves because they are less specific. Moreover, GSW paroxysm has been proposed to be the EEG manifestation of a genetic disposition and may contribute considerably to epileptogenesis in a great variety of cases [13]. The adoption of a more strict definition of GSW paroxysm has resulted in a much lower frequency in this study (7.5%) than in previous studies [3, 4, 15], although the frequency in this study is quite similar to that (7.0%) found in the siblings of SW-positive probands using a strict definition of GSW paroxysm [9, 12].

Sex of Offspring and Parent

Offspring-related factors to be considered include the sex of the offspring, whether they have a mother or a father with epilepsy, the number of EEG examinations, and the age at the time of the EEG examinations. A tendency to a higher frequency of specific EEG abnormalities in daughters and in offspring of mothers with epilepsy has been mentioned in the literature [3, 4, 22]. A more pronounced difference has been found in this and previous studies [3, 4] between sons and daughters than between offspring of affected fathers and offspring of affected mothers. However, these findings are in contrast to those of Tsuboi [22]. When both factors are combined, however, in the present study daughters of women with epilepsy have the highest frequency of GSW paroxysms, which is consistent with Tsuboi's findings [22], and next highest frequency is in daughters of men with epilepsy. There is no difference between sons of men and women with epilepsy (Table 4). By contrast Tsuboi [22] reported the second highest frequency to be in sons of women with epilepsy but no difference between children of epileptic fathers.

Number of EEG Examinations

There was no significant difference in the average number of EEG examinations between sons (2.4 EEGs) and daughters (2.6 EEGs) or between offspring of men with epilepsy (2.4 EEGs) and offspring of women with epilepsy (2.5 EEGs) in this study. The frequencies of EEG examination in sons and daughters of women with epilepsy were the same (average 2.5 EEGs). Daughters of men with epilepsy (2.6 EEGs) were examined slightly more frequently than sons of men (2.2 EEGs) and women with epilepsy (2.5 EEGs), but the differences are not statistically significant. As far as the number of EEG examinations is concerned, around a half (53.6%) of the offspring received only one EEG examination. Many more sons of men with epilepsy (63%) than of women with epilepsy (48.5%) received only one EEG examination ($\chi^2 = 3.99$, $p < 0.05$). However, there was no significant difference in the number receiving only one examination between daughters of men with epilepsy (53.2%) and sons of women with epilepsy (48.5%). Therefore, the contrasting findings with regards the frequency of GSW paroxysms in daughters of men with epilepsy and sons of women with epilepsy in this study and Tsuboi's study seem not to be related to the numbers of EEG examination.

Age at the Time of EEG Examination

The frequency of GSW paroxysms increases sharply with age, especially in daughters (Fig. 1). Continuation of EEG examinations up to the age of 24, or even better up to 29, would be needed to demonstrate the expected decline of the frequency of GSW paroxysms after the age of 16 [17, 18]. The higher frequency of GSW paroxysms in daughters than sons might not be due to the influence of age at the time of EEG examination, because the age distributions are quite simi-

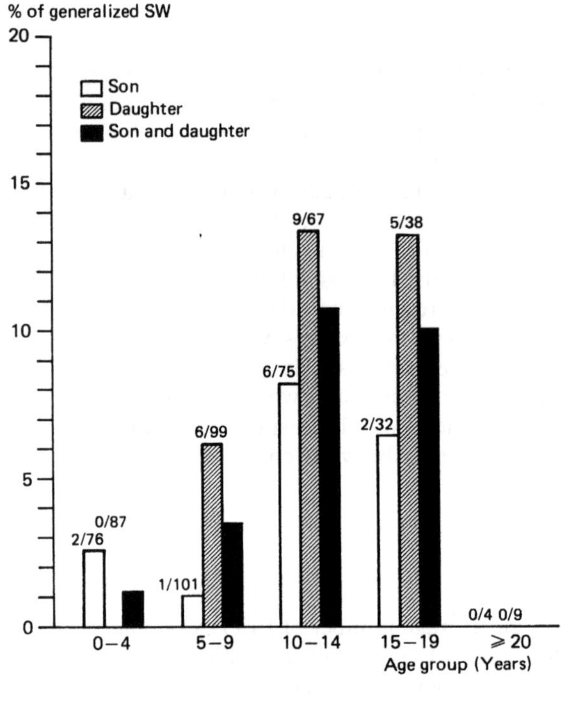

Fig. 1. Age-specific frequency of the first documentation of generalized spike and wave (*SW*) paroxysm in EEGs of sons and daughters with one epileptic parent

lar. Moreover, despite the fact of many more offspring of women with epilepsy (41.6%) than of men with epilepsy (19.1%) being examined at under 5 years of age ($\chi^2 = 56.86$, $p < 0.001$), the frequency of GSW paroxysm is still higher in offspring of women with epilepsy. The significant difference ($\chi^2 = 24.17$, $p < 0.001$) between sons of women with epilepsy (40.1%) and daughters of men with epilepsy (20.9%) in the numbers examined at less than 5 years of age might contribute to the lower frequency of GSW paroxysm found in this study in sons of women with epilepsy. Consequently, the age at EEG examination plays an important role in the detection of specific EEG abnormalities. This factor should always be considered in comparisons of the frequency of GSW paroxysm.

Types of Epilepsy and Seizure in Parent

As far as the proband is concerned, the most important factor is the type of epilepsy and seizure. The frequency of GSW paroxysms with different types of epilepsy and seizure is listed in Table 6. In accordance with other reports [4, 15, 22], offspring of probands with generalized epilepsy have a higher frequency of specific EEG abnormalities than those of probands with focal epilepsy. The highest frequency (13.8%) of GSW paroxysm is found in offspring of parents with pyknoleptic absence seizures. Interestingly, Matthes and Weber [16] and Gerken and Doose [12] have reported frequencies of GSW paroxysms of 11% and 7.5% in

Table 6. Frequency of generalized spike and wave (GSW) paroxysm in the offspring and type of epilepsy and seizure in parents

Type of epilepsy and seizure	Offspring		
	Total	With GSW	
		n	%
Generalized epilepsy	252	23	9.1
Pyknoleptic absences	58	8	13.8
Nonpyknoleptic absences	56	6	10.7
Impulsive petit mal	46	3	6.5
GTCS	87	6	6.9
Focal epilepsy	152	8	5.3

the siblings of probands with absence seizures and generalized 3/s SW paroxysms in the EEG.

Clinical Course and Implications

Serial EEGs from at least two EEG examinations among 21 GSW-positive descendants show the evolution of GSW paroxysm with time. In 12 cases (57.1%) GSW paroxysm did not reappear in the follow-up EEGs over a period of 2–8 years. In one case GSW reappeared in the fifth EEG examination at the age of 7 years. Recurrence of GSW paroxysms was found in eight cases (38.1%) Of these, four cases had persistent GSW paroxysms after their first appearance. However, the number of GSW paroxysms in successive EEGs tended to decrease with increasing age. In the other four children GSW paroxysms tended to appear irregularly.

Seizures (one child with neonatal seizures, two children with febrile seizures) and epilepsy (one child with febrile seizure and subsequently pyknoleptic absences and grand mal) were reported in four of 12 children in whom GSW paroxysms did not recur. In one child with juvenile myoclonic epilepsy GSW paroxysm appeared and disappeared in serial EEGs. In total, five of these 21 GSW-positive descendants who had at least two EEG examinations experienced clinical seizures or epilepsy. Of the other 10 GSW-positive descendants who were only examined once, one had clinical manifestations of epilepsy. Consequently, around one-fifth (six out of 31 cases, that is 19.4%) of GSW-positive descendants suffered epileptic seizures or epilepsy. Without considering the EEG examination, the risk of occurrence of epilepsy among offspring of epileptic patients is 4.6% in our study [2]. Among the 414 descendants who had at least one EEG examination, the risk of occurrence of epilepsy is 4.8% (20 out of 414 children). Taking into account the EEG findings, the risk of occurrence of epilepsy among offspring without GSW paroxysms is 4.4% (17 out of 383 children) and as high as 9.7% (three out of 31 children) in those children with GSW paroxysms in the EEG. Of the 31 children with GSW paroxysms, three had epilepsy and another three had neonatal (one child) or febrile seizures (two children). Of GSW-positive descendants, 80.6% (25 out of 31 cases) had no epileptic seizure or epilepsy. Thus, in this study, even if GSW paroxysms were seen in the EEG, around four-fifths of children with one epileptic parent had not suffered from seizure or epilepsy by the time of their last EEG.

GSW paroxysm is a genetic hallmark expressed in the EEG and may indicate a benign course of disease because it tends to disappear or to decrease in frequency in serial follow-up EEGs. Matthes and Weber have also reported comparable experiences [16]. From another viewpoint, the risk of seizure or epilepsy in offspring with GSW paroxysms is about two times higher than among those without GSW paroxysms. Moreover, specific EEG abnormalities can certainly precede the manifestation of seizures and epilepsy [7, 27]. Consequently, for genetic counseling, the question is raised, which factors may be related to the clinical manifestation of seizures or epilepsy in the descendants of epileptic patients, particularly those with GSW paroxysms. To answer this question, a prospective study is needed to evaluate the role of the factors acting as triggers to seizure manifestation [21]. This will be an important way of exploring the mechanism of triggering phenotypic manifestations of a genotype [26].

Summary and Conclusion

This study dealt with the frequency of precisely defined bilaterally synchronous generalized spike and wave (GSW) paroxysms in 414 offspring of 250 families with one epileptic parent. The EEG of offspring aged between 6 months and 20 years were recorded. The overall frequency of GSW paroxysms was 7.5%. They were more frequent in daughters (9.6%), in offspring of women with epilepsy (8.1%), in offspring of parents with generalized epilepsy (9,1%), and in the age group between 10 and 14 years (10.7%). The highest frequencies were found in daughters of women with epilepsy (11.3%) and in the offspring of parents with pyknoleptic absence seizures with or without grand mal (13.8%).

GSW paroxysms tended to disappear or to diminish in number spontaneously. Of the descendents with GSW paroxysms, three (9.7%) had neonatal or febrile seizures and another three (9.7%) had epilepsy. Of the GSW-positive descendants, 80.6% had had neither epileptic seizures nor epilepsy by the time of the last EEG examination. To elucidate the clinical manifestation of epileptic seizures or epilepsy in offspring with GSW paroxysms in the EEG, the whole sample should be studied in serial EEG examinations until the age of around 25 or even 30 and with special attention to any trigger factors related to seizure manifestation. In this way we may be able to understand the interaction of genetic and environmental factors in the clinical manifestation of seizures and epilepsy.

References

1. Andermann E, Dansky L, Andermann F, Metrakos JD, Metrakos K (1982) EEG in children of epileptic parents: findings and implications. In: Janz D, Bossi L, Dam M, Helge H, Richens A, Schmidt D (eds) Epilepsy, pregnancy and the child. Raven, New York, pp 457–467
2. Beck-Mannagetta G et al. (this volume, pp 119–126)
3. Benninger CK, Matthis P, Scheffner D (1982) EEG findings in children of epileptic parents. In: Anderson VE, Hauser WA, Penry JK, Sing CF (eds) Genetic basis of the epilepsies. Raven, New York, pp 95–99
4. Benninger C, Lipinski C, Matthis P, Scheffner D (1983) EEG Befunde bei Kindern epileptischer Eltern. In: Remschmidt H, Rentz R, Jungmann J (eds) Epilepsie 1981. Thieme, Stuttgart, pp 118–122
5. Bray PF, Wiser WC (1964) Evidence for a genetic etiology of temporal-central abnormalities in focal epilepsy. N Engl J Med 271:926–933
6. Bray PF, Wiser WC (1965) Hereditary characteristics of familial temporal-central focal epilepsy. Pediatrics 36:207–211
7. Cavazzuti GB, Cappella L, Nalin A (1980) Longitudinal study of epileptiform EEG patterns in normal children. Epilepsia 21:43–55
8. Doose H, Gerken H, Völzke E (1972) On the genetics of EEG-anomalies in childhood. I. Abnormal theta rhythms. Neuropädiatrie 3:386–401
9. Doose H, Gerken H, Horstmann T, Völzke E (1973) Genetic factors in spike wave absences. Epilepsia 14:57–75
10. Doose H, Gerken H (1973) On the genetics of EEG-anomalies in childhood. IV. Photoconvulsive reaction. Neuropädiatrie 4:162–171
11. Eeg-Olofsson O, Petersen I, Selden U (1971) The development of the electroencephalogramm in normal children from the age of 1 through 15 years: paroxysmal activity. Neuropädiatrie 2:375–404
12. Gerken H, Doose H (1973) On the genetics of EEG-anomalies in childhood. III. Spikes and waves. Neuropädiatrie 4:88–97
13. Gloor P, Metrakos J, Metrakos K, Andermann E, van Gelder N (1982) Neurophysiological, genetic and biochemical nature of the epileptic diathesis. In: Broughton RJ (ed) Henri Gastaut and the Marseilles school's contribution to the neurosciences. Electroencephalogr Clin Neurophysiol [suppl] 35:45–56
14. Kellaway P, Frost JD Jr, Crawley JW (1980) Time modulation of spike-and-wave activity in generalized epilepsy. Ann Neurol 8:491–500
15. Lipinski C, Benninger C, Janz D, Scheffner D, Seminario P, Stolzis L (1976) Historical data and EEG findings in children of epileptic and nonepileptic parents. In: Janz D (ed) Epileptology. Thieme, Stuttgart, pp 29–32
16. Matthes A, Weber H (1968) Klinische und elektroenzephalographische Familienuntersuchungen bei Pyknolepsien. Dtsch Med Wochenschr 93:429–435
17. Metrakos K, Metrakos JD (1961) Genetics of convulsive disorders. II. Genetic and electroencephalographic studies in centrencephalic epilepsy. Neurology 11:474–483
18. Metrakos K, Metrakos JD (1974) Genetics of epilepsy. In: Vinken PJ, Bruyn GW (eds) Handbook of clinical neurology, vol 15. North-Holland, Amsterdam, pp 429–439
19. Rabending G, Klepel H (1970) Fotokonvulsivreaktion und Fotomyoklonus: Altersabhängige genetisch determinierte Varianten der gesteigerten Fotosensibilität. Neuropädiatrie 2:164–172
20. Scheffner D (1982) EEG in offspring (newborns, infants and children) of epileptic parents: a review. In: Janz D, Bossi L, Dam M, Helge H, Richens A, Schmidt D (eds) Epilepsy, pregnancy and the child. Raven, New York, pp 449–455
21. Taylor DC, Bower BD (1971) Prevention in epileptic disorders. Lancet II:1136–1138
22. Tsuboi T (1982) Incidence of EEG abnormality among offspring of epileptic patients. In: Janz D, Bossi L, Dam M, Helge H, Richens A, Schmidt D (eds) Epilepsy, pregnancy, and the child. Raven, New York, pp 483–486
23. Tsuboi T (1986) Seizures of childhood. Acta Neurol Scand 74 [Suppl 110]:170–180

24. Tsuboi T, Christian W (1973) On the genetics of the primary generalized epilepsy with sporadic myoclonias of impulsive petit mal type. A clinical and electroencephalographic study of 399 probands. Humangenetik 19:155–182
25. Tsuboi T, Endo S (1977) Incidence of seizures and EEG abnormalities among offspring of epileptic patients. Humangenetik 36:173–189
26. Tsuboi T, Okada S (1985) The genetics of epilepsy. In: Sakai T, Tsuboi T (eds) Genetic aspects of human behavior. Igeku-Shoin, Tokyo, pp 113–127
27. Zivin L, Ajmone Marsan C (1968) Incidence and prognostic significance of "epileptiform" activity in the EEG of non-epileptic subjects. Brain 91:751–778

Febrile Convulsions, Epileptic Seizures and EEG Abnormalities in Offspring of Epileptic Mothers

M. L. Granström [1], E. Gaily [1], G. Beck-Mannagetta [2], and H. Klepel [3]

Introduction

In different studies the prevalence rates of febrile convulsions varied from 0.1% to 15%, and the rates of epileptic seizures in childhood from 0.1% to 3.1% [11]. A British cohort study of 13135 children found a cumulative incidence of 2.3% for febrile convulsions up to 5 years of age [12]. Tsuboi [11] observed a prevalence of 8.3% for febrile convulsions and 0.9% for afebrile convulsions in a cohort study of 17044 Japanese children followed up to the age of 3 years. A 0.41% cumulative incidence of epilepsy up to 11 years of age was observed in a British study [6]. According to Hauser and Kurland [6] the prevalence of epilepsy in the age group from birth to 9 years is 0.28%.

An increased risk of epilepsy among the offspring of epileptic mothers has been found in several studies [1, 4, 10]. In Annegers' study [1], an increased risk of both epilepsy and febrile convulsions was observed. Paroxysmal EEG abnormalities have been registered five to ten times more frequently than expected in children of epileptic mothers [9, 10].

This report presents the results of three prospective collaborative studies on the occurrence of febrile convulsions, epileptic seizures, and EEG abnormalities in children of epileptic mothers.

Material and Methods

The subjects of the three collaborative studies were 365 children of 316 epileptic mothers (E group) and 320 control children of 301 mothers (Table 1). The numbers of children in these studies by follow-up time are presented in Table 2. Waking and sleeping EEG recordings were obtained at least once in 96% of E-group children and 79% of controls at the age of 4–6 years (Table 2).

E-group mothers were recruited into the study during pregnancy. They were divided into two main groups by seizure type (Table 3) according to the international classification [3]. The control group comprised children born of nonepileptic mothers at the same obstetric hospitals.

[1] Children's Castle Hospital, Lastenlinnantie 2, SF-00250 Helsinki.
[2] Neurologische Abteilung, Universitätsklinikum Rudolf Virchow, Freie Universität Berlin, Spandauer Damm 130, D-1000 Berlin 19.
[3] Klinik für Neurologie und Psychiatrie, Medizinische Akademie, Leipziger Str. 44, DDR-3090 Magdeburg.

Genetics of the Epilepsies
Beck-Mannagetta et al. (Eds.)

Table 1. Numbers of children and mothers in the collaborative studies

Group	Study	Children	Mothers
Epileptic	Helsinki	136	125
Epileptic	West Berlin	127	102
Epileptic	Magdeburg	102	91
Total epileptic group		365	316
Control	Helsinki	145	145
Control	West Berlin	91	83
Control	Magdeburg	84	73
Total control group		320	301

Table 2. Numbers of children followed up to the ages of 18–24 months and 4–6 years in the collaborative studies

Group	Study	Child follow-up		EEG at 4–6 years
		18–24 months	4–6 years	
Epileptic	Helsinki	136	125	116
Epileptic	West Berlin	99	57	57
Epileptic	Magdeburg	82	54	54
Total epileptic group		317	236	227
Control	Helsinki	145	105	67
Control	West Berlin	59	28	28
Control	Magdeburg	60	49	49
Total control group		264	182	144

Table 3. Maternal seizure type in the collaborative studies

Study	Generalized	Partial	Unclassified
Helsinki	90 (66%)	44 (32%)	2
West Berlin	87 (69%)	40 (31%)	
Magdeburg	71 (70%)	31 (30%)	
Total	248 (68%)	115 (31%)	2

Of the children of mothers with generalized seizures, 219 were followed up to 18–24 months and 162 to 4–6 years of age. 90 children of mothers with partial seizures were followed to 18–24 months and 72 to 4–6 years. The two children whose mother had unclassified seizures were followed up to 4–6 years. EEG recordings were made at 4–6 years of age in 156 children of mothers with generalized seizures, in 69 children whose mothers had partial seizures, and in both of the children whose mother's seizures were unclassified.

Results

By the age of 18–24 months, 15 (4.7%) E-group children and 9 (3.4%) controls had febrile convulsions at least once. One child in the control group and one in the E-group followed up to 4–6 years experienced febrile convulsions after the age of 24 months (Table 4). None of the mothers whose children had febrile convulsions had a history of febrile convulsions herself. The seizure type of the mothers of children with febrile convulsions was generalized in 11 cases (73.3%) and partial with or without secondary generalization in four cases (26.5%).

Epileptic seizures occurred in five (1.6%) E-group children up to the age of 18–24 months, and in one more at the age of 4 years. The cumulative incidence of epileptic seizures in the offspring is presented in Table 5. In one epileptic child, febrile convulsions preceded the onset of epilepsy. None of the control children experienced epileptic seizures.

Generalized spike waves and sharp and slow waves (SSW) including photosensitivity were observed significantly more often in the EEG recordings of E-group children than in those of control children (Table 6). Focal slow waves were equally common in both groups. Of the children of mothers with generalized seizures, 16.7% had SSWs in their EEG recordings, as did 16.0% of the children of mothers with partial seizures and both children of the mother with unclassified

Table 4. Cumulative incidence of febrile convulsions up to the age of 4–6 years

Group	Study	18–24 months	4–6 years
Epileptic	Helsinki	4/136 (2.9%)	5/125 (4.0%)
Epileptic	West Berlin	5/ 99 (5.1%)	2/ 57 (3.5%)
Epileptic	Magdeburg	6/ 82 (7.3%)	4/ 54 (7.4%)
Total epileptic group		15/317 (4.7%)	11/236 (4.7%)
Control	Helsinki	4/145 (2.8%)	3/105 (2.9%)
Control	West Berlin	4/ 59 (8.5%)	3/ 28 (10.7%)
Control	Magdeburg	1/ 60 (1.7%)	1/ 49 (2.0%)
Total control group		9/264 (3.4%)	7/182 (3.8%)

Table 5. Cumulative incidence of epileptic seizures up to the ages of 18–24 months and 4–6 years

Group	Study	18–24 months	4–6 years
Epileptic	Helsinki	1 /136 (0.7%)	2/125 (1.6%)
Epileptic	West Berlin	1 / 99 (1.0%)	1/ 57 (1.8%)
Epileptic	Magdeburg	3 / 82 (3.1%)	1/ 54 (1.9%)
Total epileptic group		5[a]/317 (1.6%)	4/236 (1.7%)
Total control group		0	0

[a] Maternal seizure type was generalized in two cases, partial in two cases and unclassified in one case.

Table 6. EEG findings at the age of 4–6 years

Group	Study	Total	EEG with SSW		EEG with focal slow waves	
			n	%	*n*	%
Epileptic	Helsinki	116	23	(19.8)	2	(1.7)
Epileptic	West Berlin	57	10	(17.5)	2	(3.5)
Epileptic	Magdeburg	54	6	(11.1)	3	(5.6)
Total epileptic group		227	39	(17.2)[a]	7	(3.1)
Control	Helsinki	67	4	(6.0)	2	(3.0)
Control	West Berlin	26	1	(3.8)	1	(3.8)
Control	Magdeburg	49	1	(2.0)	0	0
Total control group		142	6	(4.2)[a]	3	(2.1)

[a] For total epileptic group versus total control group, $P<0.01$.

seizures. Focal slow waves were observed in the EEG recordings of 3.8% of children whose mothers had generalized seizures and in 1.4% of children whose mothers had partial seizures.

Febrile convulsions were about as common among the children who had paroxysmal EEG findings (3/55, 5.5%) as in the total E-group (4.7%) and control group (3.8%). The only child with a history of both febrile convulsions and subsequent epilepsy had SSWs in her EEG recording at the age of 4–6 years.

Altogether four of the 17 children (23.5%) with febrile convulsions showed paroxysmal EEG abnormalities at the age of 4–6 years. Three of the four children with epileptic seizures had an abnormal EEG. The EEG of the fourth epileptic child was normal.

The mothers of the children with febrile convulsions and/or epilepsy were not younger at the onset of their epilepsy than the other epileptic mothers.

Discussion

According to the results of this prospective study, the risk of febrile convulsions is not significantly increased in children of epileptic mothers. This is in agreement with some earlier observations [4, 10], but differs from the report of Annegers et al. [1]. This finding indicates that the inheritance of febrile convulsions is independent of the inheritance of epilepsy. From our data, we can make no estimation of the degree of inherited risk of febrile convulsions, because we do not have complete family histories of all of the children in the study. There were two sibling pairs with febrile convulsions in this material but none of the mothers whose children had febrile convulsions had experienced febrile convulsions herself as a child.

The risk of epilepsy was higher than expected in children of epileptic mothers, even within this short follow-up period; this agrees with earlier reports [1, 4, 10]. In order to estimate the degree of risk more comprehensively, one would have to follow the children up to adult age. According to our figures in contrast to earlier studies [4, 7, 10], the occurrence of epilepsy in offspring was not associated with maternal seizure type or age at onset of epileptic seizures. The present study material is, however, too limited to make a reliable estimation.

The risk of epilepsy has been found to be increased in children with febrile convulsions in general, particularly in children with other neurological symptoms or prolonged or atypical febrile seizures [2]. In children with febrile convulsions, the risk of subsequent epilepsy has been observed to be higher if the child has family members with either epilepsy or febrile convulsions [2, 7]. Apparently, in some cases, epilepsy presents with febrile convulsions; this risk is increased in the offspring of epileptic mothers in this study. However, in epidemiological studies the proportion of this kind of febrile convulsions is probably too small to affect the general risk of febrile seizures in the children of epileptic mothers.

It has been suggested that paroxysmal EEG abnormalities, especially spikes and waves, reflect predisposition to seizures. The frequency of such EEG findings was considerably higher in children of epileptic mothers than in controls, as reported earlier [9]. In our study, EEG abnormalities were associated with epilepsy in offspring but not with febrile convulsions. Due to the short follow-up period in our study, the predictive value of paroxysmal EEG abnormalities at 4–6 years with regard to the risk of epilepsy at a later age remains undetermined.

References

1. Annegers JF, Hauser WA, Elveback LR, Anderson VE, Kurland LT (1976) Seizure disorders in offspring of parents with a history of seizures – a maternal-paternal difference? Epilepsia 17:1–9
2. Annegers JF, Hauser WA, Elveback LR, Kurland LT (1979) The risk of epilepsy following febrile convulsions. Neurology 29:297–303
3. Commission on Classification and Terminology of the International League Against Epilepsy (1981) Proposal for revised clinical and electroencephalographic classification of epileptic seizures. Epilepsia 22:489–501
4. Beck-Mannagetta G, Janz D, Lipinski D (1982) Febrile convulsions in children of epileptic parents: A retrospective study. In: Janz D et al. (eds) Epilepsy, pregnancy and the child. Raven, New York, pp 521–526
5. Janz D, Beck-Mannagetta G, Scheffner D, Scholz G (1982) Epilepsy in children of epileptic parents. In: Janz D et al. (eds) Epilepsy, pregnancy, and the child. Raven, New York, pp 527–534
6. Hauser WA, Kurland LT (1975) The epidemiology of epilepsy in Rochester, Minnesota, 1935 through 1967. Epilepsia 16:1–66
7. Nelson KB, Ellenberg JH (1978) Prognosis in children with febrile seizures. Pediatrics 61:720–727
8. Ross EM, Peckham CS, West PB, Butler NR (1980) Epilepsy in childhood: Findings from the National Child Developmental Study. Br Med J:207–210
9. Scheffner D (1982) EEG in offspring (newborn, infants and children) of epileptic parents: A review. In: Janz D et al. (eds) Epilepsy, pregnancy and the child. Raven, New York, pp 449–455
10. Tsuboi T, Endo S (1977) Incidence of seizures and EEG abnormalities among offspring of epileptic patients. Hum Genet 36:173–189
11. Tsuboi T (1984) Epidemiology of febrile and afebrile convulsions in children in Japan. Neurology 34:175–181
12. Verity CM, Butler NR, Golding J (1985) Febrile convulsions in a national cohort followed up from birth. I. Prevalence and recurrence in the first five years of life. Br Med J 290:1307–1310

Special Methods

Twin Studies in Epilepsy

V. E. Anderson [1], K. J. Wilcox [1], S. S. Rich [2], I. E. Leppik [3], and W. A. Hauser [4]

A number of twin studies of epilepsy, both larger series and individual case studies, have been reported. These have shown clearly that both genetic and environmental factors are involved, but they have not contributed significantly to the understanding of basic mechanisms. Meanwhile, there has been rapid progress in the neurosciences, with respect to brain structure and function, brain imaging, neurophysiology, and biochemistry at the cellular and molecular levels [8, 27]. New questions have arisen and new methods for study have been developed.

The time has come for a new and more focused use of twin methods. Some of the existing data sets can be reanalyzed. New samples can be collected in preparation for studies using the new methods for assessment. Such plans, however, must take into account both the unique advantages and the limitations of twin methods.

The Value of Twin Studies

The study of twins has been applied to the investigation of a number of medical problems, in an effort to determine the relative contributions of genetic and environmental factors [5, 14]. Methods have been developed that recognize the special biological and statistical problems associated with twin studies [1, 2, 33, 34].

In terms of the ascertainment of cases, twin studies include population-based surveys (identifying twins from birth records), clinic-based series (having good clinical data, but usually biased in the direction of more severe and chronic cases), and case reports of a single twin pair. Each approach is useful, but they do not answer the same questions.

In terms of family structure, the simplest studies are limited to the twin pairs alone, while others include the extended family. It has been shown by simulation studies that the twin-family design needs only a fraction of the sample size required by the classical twin design [21]. The study of offspring of twins provides even more data and permits the answering of more complex questions [22, 20].

[1] Department of Genetics and Cell Biology, Dight Laboratories, University of Minnesota, 400 Church Street S. E., Minneapolis, MN 55455, USA.
[2] Department of Laboratory Medicine and Pathology, Box 511 Mayo, University of Minnesota, Hospital and Clinic, 500 Harvard Street S. E., Minneapolis, MN 55455, USA.
[3] Department of Neurology, Box 389 Mayo, University of Minnesota, Hospital and Clinic, 500 Harvard Street S. E., Minneapolis, MN 55455, USA.
[4] G. H. Sergievsky Center, Columbia University, 630 West 168th Street, New York, NY 10032, USA.

Genetics of the Epilepsies
Beck-Mannagetta et al. (Eds.)

When longitudinal data are available, twin methods are well-suited for the analysis of developmental (age-related) changes, with particular attention given to gene-environment interaction [9]. It is not always valid to generalize from a twin series to the general single-born population, however. The risk of congenital malformations, for example, is higher in twins than it is in the general population [26].

Concordance for Epilepsy

The concordance rate for epilepsy is considerably higher in monozygotic (MZ) than in dizygotic (DZ) pairs in most of the published studies [23]. Combining six of the major studies, the concordance rate for epilepsy is 60% for MZ pairs and 13% for DZ pairs [35].

The largest series of twins identified through clinical practice is the one studied by Lennox and Lennox [17]. When analysis is limited to chronic seizures (Table 1), the concordance is 44% for MZ pairs and 7% for DZ pairs ($\chi^2 = 40.6$, $p < 0.001$). In twins with clinical data suggesting a brain lesion in the index case, concordance was seen in 11% of MZ pairs and 7% of DZ pairs ($\chi^2 = 0.3$, NS). On the other hand, when the clinical information favored an intact brain, concordance was seen in 33 out of 47 (70%) MZ pairs as contrasted with 3 out of 54 (6%) DZ pairs ($\chi^2 = 45.8$, $p < 0.001$).

In a smaller series, Inouye [15] identified 40 twin pairs from both outpatients and inpatients. In reanalyzing the data, we excluded a pair with ichthyosis combined with mental retardation, a pair with phenylketonuria, a pair with epiloia (tuberous sclerosis), and a pair first identified at 79 years of age. Among 24 MZ pairs, 12 (50%) were concordant for epilepsy. (In the 12 discordant MZ pairs, seven of the unaffected co-twins had an abnormal EEG.) Among 12 DZ pairs, none were concordant for epilepsy, although in one pair the co-twin had febrile seizures. (There was EEG information on eight of the DZ co-twins, and two showed an abnormal EEG.) The concordance for epilepsy in the MZ pairs (50%) is significantly different ($p < 0.01$) from that in the DZ pairs (0%).

Table 1. Epilepsy in twins

Study	MZ pairs		DZ pairs	
	Total	Concordant	Total	Concordant
Inouye [16]				
Total	26	14 (54%)	14	1 (7%)
After exclusions	24	12 (50%)	12	0
Lennox and Lennox [17]				
Total	95	59 (62%)	130	19 (15%)
Chronic only	84	37 (44%)	121	8 (7%)
Brain injured	37	4 (11%)	67	5 (7%)
Intact	47	33 (70%)	54	3 (6%)
Harvald and Hauge [13]	27	10 (37%)	100	10 (10%)

Table 2. Seizure type in twins without brain injury: Lennox and Lennox [17]

Seizure type	MZ pairs		DZ pairs	
	Total	Concordant	Total	Concordant
Grand mal (GM)	51	42 (82%)	52	8 (15%)
Petit mal (PM)	20	15 (75%)	14	0
GM and PM	13	10 (77%)	8	0
Psychomotor	13	5 (39%)	19	1 (5%)
GM and psychomotor	11	3 (27%)	10	0

The largest population-based twin study of epilepsy involved a follow-up of all twins born in Denmark in the years 1870–1910 [13]. Among the MZ pairs 37% were concordant for epilepsy, while among the DZ pairs 10% were concordant ($\chi^2 = 11.7, p < 0.001$). It may be noted that these MZ and DZ rates are not significantly different from the MZ and DZ rates in the Inouye and Lennox studies.

Lennox and Lennox [17] analyzed a number of other clinical details, including seizure type (Table 2). Here the MZ/DZ difference in concordance is more striking than in Table 1. Unfortunately, the twins with multiple seizure types are counted more than once, and it is not possible to reconstruct the data by persons rather than by seizure types. The original information is still on file in considerable detail, however, and it may be possible to reevaluate the seizure history according to current criteria and to tabulate the data by individuals.

Finally, these three studies are of the quality that might justify a follow-up of offspring to determine how many have developed seizures. This approach has been particularly effective in the case of schizophrenia, where it was found that the risk was as high for the children of the discordant (unaffected) MZ co-twins as for the children of the affected twins [4].

Febrile Convulsions

Several twin studies of febrile convulsions have been reported. Lennox-Buchthal [18, 19] analyzed the data for the Lennox twin series and found concordance for febrile convulsions to be 68% in MZ pairs, as compared with 13% in DZ pairs (Table 3). It was noted, however, that among these twins a higher proportion had a severely abnormal birth history with subsequent epilepsy than did the population-based series studied in Denmark by Frantzen et al. [11]. This difference between the Lennox series (in Boston) and the Danish series may represent, in part, a selective bias toward severity and multiple seizure types in the cases referred to Dr. Lennox. There remains the possibility, however, that the perinatal risks associated with twin pregnancy and delivery may contribute somewhat to the risk of febrile convulsions.

Schiøttz-Christensen [28] searched the records for twins born in the Copenhagen area from 1950–1965. The incidence of febrile convulsions among all twin-born individuals was estimated at 3.0%. The concordance for febrile convulsions

Table 3. Febrile convulsions in twins

Study	MZ pairs		DZ pairs	
	Total	Concordant	Total	Concordant
Lennox-Buchthal [18, 19]	19	13 (68%)	46	6 (13%)
Schiøttz-Christensen [28]	26	8 (31%)	37	5 (14%)
Tsuboi and Okada [35]				
Population	9	4 (44%)	7	1 (14%)
Clinic	10	7 (70%)	7	0

was 31% in MZ pairs and 14% in DZ pairs (Table 3). This difference is not statistically significant, and the results have been cited as evidence against genetic factors. It seems more reasonable to conclude that the results were indefinite (because of the relatively small sample size) and that both genetic and nongenetic factors are involved.

The ascertainment of the probands (index cases) was so well-described in the Schiøttz-Christensen study that the "case-wise" risk of febrile convulsions could be calculated as 44% for MZ co-twins of probands and 20% for DZ co-twins. The risk of febrile convulsions in *single-born* siblings of the twin probands was 10.8%. (The rate of 14% reported in the original paper included the DZ co-twins, which does not seem appropriate). The almost two-fold difference between the risk for DZ co-twins and the risk for single-born siblings provides further evidence for the possible effect of twinning per se.

In a series of later papers some additional findings on the Danish twin cohort were reported. The risk of subsequent epilepsy was 2.6% over an 11-year follow-up period [30]. The twins with febrile convulsions did not have more indicators of birth trauma than did the unaffected co-twins [30]. However, the twins with febrile convulsions did show a tendency toward lower performance on intellectual and neurological tests [31, 29] and more often had an abnormal EEG [32] than did their unaffected co-twins.

Case Reports

Although the emphasis in this discussion has been on twin series, there are situations in which careful evaluation of one twin pair can provide critical information to test hypotheses or suggest new approaches. A few selected reports may serve to illustrate this point.

An MZ pair began having generalized convulsions at the age of 9 years. The major seizures decreased in frequency as minor seizures increased. A sensitivity to light flashes was noted early and was documented in the EEG when the twins were examined at 42 years [7]. Although the report was published in 1951, an effort to follow any offspring and other relatives might be rewarding. A similar suggestion can be made for a report in 1963 of three families which included an MZ twin pair concordant for temporal lobe epilepsy [3].

Early evidence for genetic variation in fetal susceptibility to the teratogenic effects of phenytoin came from a report of DZ twin girls who were most likely fathered by two men of different races [25]. At four years of age the twins were discordant for many features of the fetal hydantoin syndrome.

The value of testing co-twins is illustrated by the case of a 30-year-old male who became stuporous seven days after valproic acid (VPA) was added to other anti-epileptic drugs [6]. At that time the blood ammonia concentration was very high, but the patient's condition improved rapidly after the VPA was discontinued. A twin brother (said to be identical, although no evidence was presented) showed a similar marked increase of venous ammonia concentration after a single loading dose of VPA.

Most studies have shown that a family history of epilepsy is less important for partial than for generalized epilepsy. One girl developed partial seizures at 8 years, and her MZ co-twin at 11 years. Their EEGs were very similar, showing focal right centrotemporal epileptiform abnormalities and generalized bisynchronous 3 to 3½ cps spike-and-wave discharges with occasional right-sided dominance [15]. A longitudinal follow-up of this pair and examination of other relatives would be warranted.

Twins in the Minnesota Comprehensive Epilepsy Program

Our genetics and epidemiology sample has identified 1046 seizure patients in an incidence sample (limited to recently diagnosed cases from any cause and at any age). This sample includes 28 (2.7%) who are twin-born. In order to estimate an expected number, an essential distinction must be made: About 1% of pregnancies will produce twins, but about 2% of children will be twin-born.

Among all reported births in the United States between 1928 and 1949, 1.108% of pregnancies reaching the viable stage terminated in twin deliveries [1]. These twin pregnancies produced 2.19% of all the babies. After correcting for excess mortality in twins, the frequency of twin-born individuals was estimated to be essentially constant at 1.9% from the first year of life to age 25.

The expected number of twin-born in our sample thus would be 19.9 as compared with the 28 observed (a difference which is not significant, using the Poisson distribution). In four of the 28 pairs the co-twin is deceased. Only two of the 28 have an affected co-twin (both pairs DZ), illustrating the difficulty of recruiting a sufficient number of twins for study using systematic sampling.

As a basis for biochemical studies we have adopted the use of multisib families [12]. From a variety of sources we identified an additional 18 twin pairs, of which 5 are concordant for seizures. Because of the selection bias involved, such twin pairs are useless for estimating population parameters (such as concordance rates), but they should be essentially unbiased for biochemical analysis. Preliminary data for two twin pairs will be presented, mainly to illustrate the approach.

Blood typing of twins A and B indicated that they are a MZ pair. Both have been evaluated extensively with video monitoring, and a summary of the findings is shown in Table 4. The seizure types and EEG patterns are similar, although Twin A has been more seriously affected and has shown greater variability in sei-

Table 4. Clinical data for twins *A* and *B*

	Twin *A*	Twin *B*
Birth (March 10, 1958)	Normal	Breech
Development	Delayed	Delayed
IQ	64	66
Epilepsy	Primary generalized	Primary generalized
Seizures	Simple absence (age 5) Complex absence Atonic Tonic-clonic Myoclonic activity	Simple absence (age 5) Tonic-clonic
EEG	3/s generalized spike and wave	3/s generalized spike and wave
Dermatoglyphics	Abnormal	Abnormal
Other	Hyperthyroid	Hyperthyroid
Seizure control	Refractory	Controlled

Table 5. Clinical data for twins *C* and *D*

	Twin *C*	Twin *D*
Birth (July 6, 1950)	Normal	Normal
Epilepsy	Primary generalized	Primary generalized
Seizures	Absence (Age 16) Tonic-clonic (Age 26)	Absence (Age 14) Tonic-clonic (Age 17)
EEG	Generalized spike and wave Diffuse slowing	Generalized spike and wave Diffuse slowing Photomyoclonic response
Other	Learning difficulty Cholecystectomy	Learning difficulty Migraine

zure manifestation. Both twins were hyperthyroid and both had a partial thyroidectomy. No seizures have been reported for their parents and their three siblings.

Both twins show bilateral clinodactyly of the fifth finger and both have abnormal dermatoglyphics. (The latter includes bilateral transitional palmar creases, elevated axial triradii, reduced *atd* angles, and complex thenar patterns. Both have nine ulnar loops and one arch pattern of the fingers.) The dermatoglyphic findings appeared intriguing until we learned that a healthy sister without seizures has similar findings. Studies of other family members are under way.

Twins C and D are probably MZ, although testing has not been completed. Their seizure types and EEG patterns are strikingly similar (Table 5). They have an older sister with tonic-clonic seizures, and two younger sisters, both with recurrent seizures of unspecified type (Fig. 1). Both of the twins have children, and one of the children has developed absence seizures.

Biochemical studies of both of these familes have been initiated. In Fig. 2 the taurine excretion levels of the four twins are compared with the results from the earlier study [12]. In Figs. 1 and 3 the plasma haptoglobin levels are shown

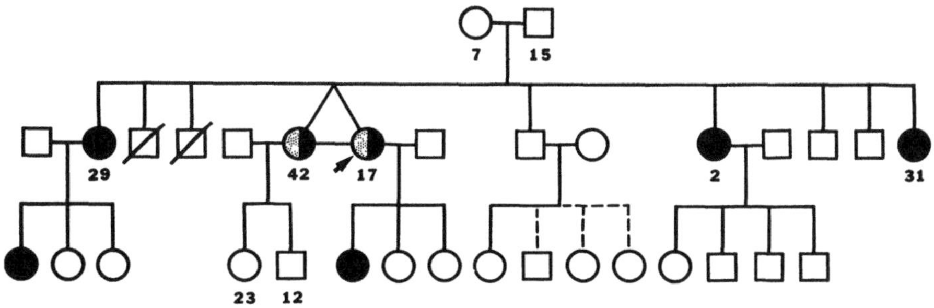

Fig. 1. Pedigree of the kindred including Twins C and D. The *dotted lines* indicate adoption. Plasma haptoglobin values (mg %) are shown for those members tested (see reference [24] for methods)

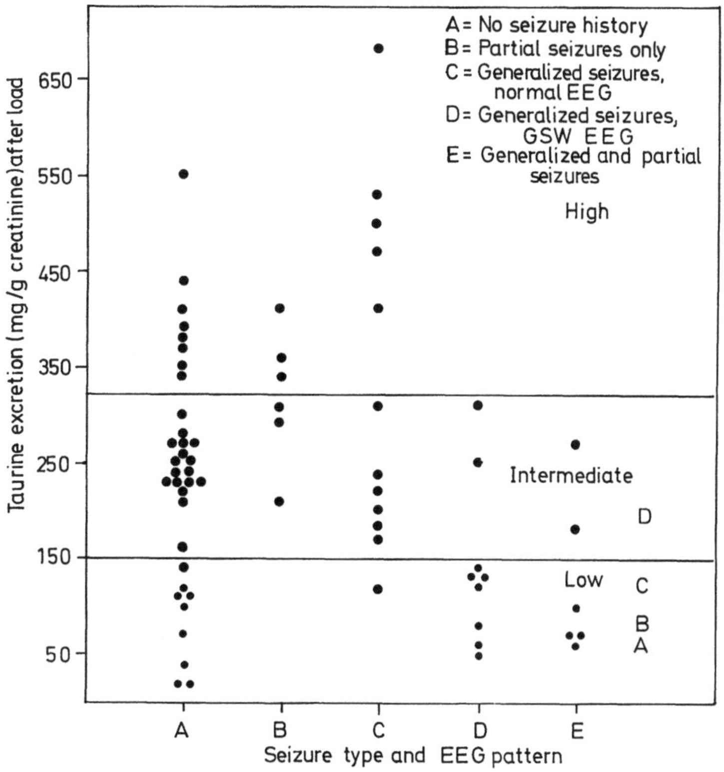

Fig. 2. The distribution of taurine excretion levels in Twins A, B, C, and D compared with subjects from families with two or more siblings affected with seizures. (Modified from [12])

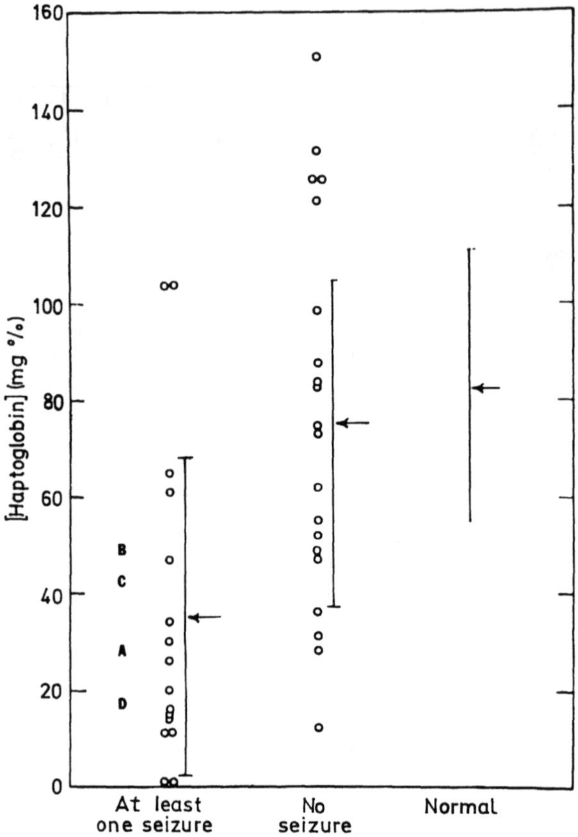

Fig. 3. The distribution of plasma haptoglobin values (*mg %*) in Twins A, B, C, and D compared with members from families with idiopathic epilepsy. (Modified from [24])

(see [24]). The study of other relatives and of other biochemical variables is under way.

Another effort to identify twins with seizures involves cooperation with the Minnesota Twin Registry (directed by David Lykken). Currently the registry has located twins born in Minnesota in the years 1936, 1937, 1949, 1954, and 1955. Among 1191 same-sex pairs in which both members returned a questionnaire, there were 24 pairs with one or both reporting a history of seizures or epilepsy. These pairs are concordant for seizures, and to our surprise two pairs (thought to be MZ) have experienced reading epilepsy. One set of twins was the subject of an extensive earlier report (10).

International Twin Registry

In the epilepsy research strategy for the near future, there are two major options: (a) population-based twin series, for more accurate estimation of concordance rates, or (b) clinic-based samples, for intensive study of seizure types, EEG patterns, and biochemical variables. Although both are important, we have chosen to emphasize the latter.

This approach can be illustrated by describing what might be done with a series of twins concordant for epilepsy, but with at least one having a history of absence seizures. The MZ pairs would be expected to have a narrower range of variability in seizure type and EEG patterns than the DZ pairs. An analysis of such results should be relevant for the classification of seizures and seizure syndromes. The twin panel also could be used to test specific etiological hypotheses.

The total twin sample available for study in any city will be relatively small, however. About one out of 50 epilepsy patients will be twin-born and only about one-third of these will be members of MZ pairs. Only a small fraction of pairs will be concordant for epilepsy. Therefore, broad collaboration will be required, and to this end an International Twin Registry has been established [37]. This registry is designed to bring research investigators into contact with those who have the necessary clinical samples.

Attention to twins is recommended for any epilepsy clinic, whether or not broader collaboration is intended. The following steps are suggested:

1. Ask all patients whether or not they are twin born, and maintain a central list of those who are twins.
2. While reviewing the EEGs, record the presence of the EEG variants described by Vogel [36].
3. Consider the possibility that clinical information about the co-twin might assist in the diagnosis and/or treatment of the present patient.
4. From time to time, review the records of twins to determine if any seem unique enough to justify the publication of a case report.

Conclusion

Twins are an experiment of nature which can provide unique insights into the role of genetics and environment in the development of epilepsy. Among concordant pairs, a comparison of MZ and DZ twins will help to define the range of variability in seizure types and EEG patterns possible in specific syndromes. On the other hand, a careful evaluation of discordant MZ pairs may identify environmental factors which account for the development of epilepsy in one member of a pair of twins with identical genotypes.

References

1. Allen G (1955) Comments on the analysis of twin samples. Acta Genet Med Gemellol 4:143–160
2. Allen G (1965) Twin research: problems and prospects. Prog Med Genet 4:242–269
3. Barslund I, Danielsen J (1963) Temporal epilepsy in monozygotic twins. Epilepsia 4:138–150
4. Bertelsen A, Gottesman II (1986) Offspring of twin pairs discordant for psychiatric illness. Paper presented at the Vth international congress twin studies, Sept 15–19, Amsterdam

5. Cameron AH, Edwards JH, Derom R, Thiery M, Boelaert R (1983) The value of twin surveys in the study of malformations. Eur J Obstet Gynecol Reprod Biol 14:347–356
6. Campostrini R, Zaccara G, Rossi L, Paganini M, Dorigotti A, Zappoli R (1985) Valproate-induced hyperammonaemia in two epileptic identical twins. J Neurol 232:167–168
7. Daly D, Bickford RG (1951) Electroencephalographic studies of identical twins with photo-epilepsy. EEG Clin Neurophysiol 3:245–249
8. Delgado-Escueta AV, Ward AA Jr, Woodbury DM, Porter RJ (eds) (1986) Advances in neurology, vol 44. Raven, New York
9. Eaves LJ (1982) The utility of twins. In: Anderson VE, Hauser WA, Penry JK, Sing CF (eds) Genetic basis of the epilepsies. Raven, New York
10. Forster F, Daly R (1973) Reading epilepsy in identical twins. Trans Am Neurol Assoc 98:186–188
11. Frantzen E, Lennox-Buchthal M, Nygaard A, Stene J (1970) A genetic study of febrile convulsions. Neurology 20:909–917
12. Haines JL, Panter SS, Rich SS, Eaton JW, Tsai MY, Anderson VE (1986) Reduced plasma haptoglobin and urinary taurine in familial seizures identified through the multisib strategy. Am J Med Genet 24:723–734
13. Harvald B, Hauge M (1965) Hereditary factors elucidated by twin studies. In: Neel JV, Shaw MW, Schull WJ (eds) Genetics and the epidemiology of chronic diseases. Public Health Service Publication No 1163, Washington DC
14. Hrubec Z, Robinette CD (1984) The study of human twins in medical research. N Engl J Med 310:435–441
15. Hurst R, Lenn NJ (1986) Partial seizures in monozygous twins. Epilepsia 27:121–123
16. Inouye E (1960) Observations on forty twin index cases with chronic epilepsy and their co-twins. J Nerv Ment Dis 130:401–416
17. Lennox WG, Lennox MA (1960) Epilepsy and related disorders. Little, Brown, Boston
18. Lennox-Buchthal M (1971) Febrile and nocturnal convulsions in monozygotic twins. Epilepsia 12:147–156
19. Lennox-Buchthal MA (1973) Febrile convulsions. A reappraisal. EEG Clin Neurophysiol (suppl 32):1–132
20. McGue M, Rao DC, Isélius L, Russell JM (1985) Resolution of genetic and cultural inheritance in twin families by path analysis: Application to HDL cholesterol. Am J Hum Genet 37:998–1014
21. Moll PP, Sing CF (1979) Sampling strategies for the analysis of quantitative traits. In: Sing CF, Skolnick M (eds) Genetic analysis of common diseases: applications to predictive factors on coronary disease. Liss, New York
22. Nance WE, Corey LA, Boughman JA (1978) Monozygotic twin kinships: a new design for genetic and epidemiological research. In: Morton NE, Chung CS (eds) Genetic epidemiology. Academic, New York
23. Newmark ME, Penry JK (eds) (1980) Genetics of epilepsy: a review. Raven, New York
24. Panter SS, Sadrzadeh SM, Hallaway PE, Haines J, Anderson VE, Eaton JW (1985) Hypohaptoglobinemia: a possible predisposition to epilepsy. Trans Assoc Am Physicians 97:56–62
25. Phelan MC, Pellock JM, Nance WE (1982) Discordant expression of fetal hydantoin syndrome in heteropaternal dizygotic twins. N Engl J Med 307:99–101
26. Propping P, Vogel F (1976) Twin studies in medical genetics. Acta Genet Med Gemellol 25:249–258
27. Rosenberg MB, Hansen C Jr, Breakefield XO (1985) Molecular genetic approaches to neurologic and psychiatric diseases. Progr Neurobiol 24:95–140
28. Schiøttz-Christensen E (1972) Genetic factors in febrile convulsions: an investigation of 64 same-sexed twin pairs. Acta Neurol Scand 48:538–546
29. Schiøttz-Christensen E (1973 a) Neurological findings in twins discordant for febrile convulsions. Acta Neurol Scand 49:368–378
30. Schiøttz-Christensen E (1973 b) Role of birth history in the aetiology and course of febrile convulsions. A twin study. Neuropaediatrie 4:239–244
31. Schiøttz-Christensen E, Bruhn P (1973) Intelligence, behaviour and scholastic achievement subsequent to febrile convulsions: an analysis of discordant twin pairs. Develop Med Child Neurol 15:565–575

32. Schiøttz-Christensen E, Hammerberg PE (1975) EEG in twins with febrile convulsions. Follow-up on 59 pairs of the same sex. Neuropaediatrie 6:142–150
33. Smith C (1970) Heritability of liability and concordance in monozygotic twins. Ann Hum Genet 34:85–91
34. Smith C (1974) Concordance in twins: methods and interpretations. Am J Hum Genet 26:454–466
35. Tsuboi T, Okada S (1985) The genetics of epilepsy. In: Sakai T, Tsuboi T (eds) Genetic aspects of human behavior. Igaku-Shoin, Tokyo
36. Vogel F (1988) Genetic variation of the normal human EEG (this volume)
37. Those interested may write to: Epilepsy Twin Registry, Dight Laboratories, University of Minnesota, 400 Church Street S E, Minneapolis, MN 55455, USA

HLA and Epilepsy

M. DURNER [1], J. ZINGSEM [2], D. A. GREENBERG [3], T. SANDER [1], and D. JANZ [1]

Introduction

The association of HLA antigens with some specific diseases has given us the opportunity to increase our understanding of these diseases. In these diseases of unknown etiology, the condition occurs more frequently in families of affected people then in the general population. The mode of inheritance is generally unknown. Association indicates that at least part of the genetic basis lies in the HLA region. The HLA region (or MHC) is located on the short arm of chromosome 6 and is composed of the A, B, C, and D locus. Linked with these loci are several loci not involved in immunological mechanisms such as genes for complement factors (C2, Bf, C4) and enzymes (phosphoglucomutase 3, PGM3; glyoxalase 1, GLO). Furthermore, the genes for susceptibility to hemochromatosis (HFE) and congenital adrenal hyperplasia (CA21H) have been mapped to the HLA region itself.

One very important characteristic of the HLA genes is that they are highly polymorphic, i.e., several alleles exist at each locus. This makes the HLA system an ideal marker for genetic association or linkage studies. Genes are called linked when their loci are situated close to one another. When two loci are linked, there is a greater probability that genetic recombination between them will not occur during gamete formation. When recombination does not occur, the alleles at the two loci are inherited together. Linkage is detected only within families. In the general population, any two alleles at two loci that are linked are not found together more often than expected. Association, on the other hand, is a population phenomenon. Association is detected by testing whether a certain allele occurs more frequently in the population with the disease (or trait) than in the general population. Therefore, linkage studies have to be studies of the patients' families, whilst for association studies one investigates patients and control groups.

Table 1 gives a summary of all the previous studies done on HLA and epilepsy. Many syndromes have been studied, some of them very inhomogenous. The numbers of patients investigated in these studies are fairly small. We will consider several studies in detail.

[1] Neurologische Abteilung, Universitätsklinikum Rudolf Virchow, Freie Universität Berlin, Spandauer Damm 130, D-1000 Berlin 19.
[2] Blutbank, Universitätsklinikum Rudolf Virchow, Freie Universität Berlin, Spandauer Damm 130, D-1000 Berlin 19.
[3] Southwest Regional VA Epilepsy Center, Neurology Service, Wadsworth VA Medical Center, Los Angeles. Current address: Department of Psychiatry, Mt. Sinai Medical Center, 1 Gustave Levy Place, New York, NY 10029, USA.

Genetics of the Epilepsies
Beck-Mannagetta et al. (Eds.)

Table 1. HLA and epilepsy

Study	Disease	No. of patients
1976 Smeraldi et al. [14]	Lennox-Gastaut syndrome	22
1978 Howitz and Platz [7]	Epilepsy with infantile spasm	21
1978 Fontana et al. [4]	Epilepsy with IgA deficiency	19
1978 Shakir et al. [13]	Epilepsy with IgA deficiency	10
	Epilepsy without IgA deficiency	10
1979 Westphal et al. [15]	Epilepsy with myoclonic-astatic seizures	49
	Photosensitivity with seizures	63
	Photosensitivity without seizures	25
1981 Fichsel and Kessler [3]	Epilepsy with 3 Hz absence	26
1982 Eeg-Olofsson et al. [1]	Benign epilepsy of childhood	21
	Epilepsy with absences	18
	Epilepsy with TCS	9
	Epilepsy with complex partial seizures	5
1982 Monoghan et al. [10]	Cryptogenic myoclonic epilepsy	19
1983 Rivas [11]	Petit mal epilepsy	42
1985 Hafez et al. [6]	Epilepsy with absences	16
	Epilepsy with idiopathic TCS	36
1985 Eeg-Olofsson et al. [2]	Partial epilepsy	24
1987 Minev et al. [9]	Epilepsy of unknown origin	51
	Epilepsy with absence	24
1987 Gerstle de Pasquet et al. [5]	Generalized epilepsy	25
	Partial epilepsy	29

Lennox's Syndrome

From the information given in the papers one can assume that Smeraldi (1976) investigated the idiopathic and symptomatic forms of Lennox's sydrome [14], while Westphal [15] and Monoghan [10] looked at only the idiopathic form of the same syndrome. Only Smeraldi (1976) found a significant increase in the frequency of HLA-B7 in his patients (Table 2). In the patients studied by Westphal and Monoghan the distribution of HLA antigens did not differ significantly from that in the general population. However, it must be noted that there is a remarkable difference in the relative frequency of HLA-B7 in the control groups of the various studies.

Table 2. HLA-B 7 and lennox's syndrome

Study	Patients		Control
	n	%+	%+
Smeraldi et al.	22	45	10
Westphal et al.	49	18	46
Monoghan et al.	19	53	31

Absences

Another subgroup of patients, namely those with absences, has been investigated by several authors (Table 3). Fichsel and Kessler [3] found a positive association with HLA-A1 and -B8, as well as with the haplotype A1-B8. Rivas [11] also reports an increase of the haplotype A1-B8, to approximately double the frequency in the general population. Since A1 and B8 are in linkage disequilibrium, one would expect that an association with one antigen would automatically lead to an association with the other, and that the frequency of the combination of the two as haplotype would be increased as well. Eeg-Olofsson (1982) could not confirm these results [1]. In his unrelated patients, the antigen A1 and the haplotype A1-B8 were less frequent than in the general population, but not significantly. It is possible that this is due to differences in the patient populations, because Fichsel and Kessler had tried to differentiate the absences by the EEG criterion of 3-Hz spike waves. Hafez [6] observed a normal distribution of HLA-A1 and -B8 in patients with absences from Egypt, but he found a significant increase in the frequency of A9 and a decrease of A2. Fichsel and Kessler also noted a decrease in the frequency of A2, but give no numbers for this result. Nevertheless, it must be borne in mind that each increase in the frequency of one or more antigens is accompanied by a decrease in other antigens. Therefore, one cannot say for sure, without rigorous statistical analysis, that a lack of a certain antigen implies a lack of a protecting factor. Hafez also observed this association between A9 and A2 in patients with idiopathic tonic clonic seizures (TCS). It is remarkable that the frequency of HLA-A2 in his control group (37.5%) is much lower than that found in European caucasions (namely 45.3%). Nowadays HLA-A9 can be split up into Aw23 and Aw24, but nevertheless the frequency of both together is 4.5 times higher (22.7%) than in his control group (5%).

The only investigation which also concerns the Dr locus is by Minev [9]. There were no differences in the frequencies of the HLA-A, -B, and C-antigens, but

Table 3. HLA and absence

Study	Antigen	Patients		Control		Relative risk
		n	% +	*n*	% +	
Fichsel and Kessler	A1	26	52	331	28	3.0
	B8		44		19	3.0
Eeg-Olofsson et al.	A1	18	11	500	22	0.4
	B8		22		19	1.2
	A2		67		61	1.3
	A9		33		19	2.1
Hafez et al.	A1	16	25	120	15	1.8
	A8		6		5	1.2
	A2		19		37	0.4
	A9		44		5	14.7
Minev et al.	Dr5	24	58	200	27	

there was an increase of Dr5, especially in patients with absences and additional TCS.

Rolandic Epilepsy

Eeg-Olofsson studied 21 patients with benign epilepsy of childhood with centro temporal spikes, nine patients with TCS, and five patients with complex partial seizures [1]. He found no statistical deviation from the normal HLA distribution, but a statistically significant decrease in the frequency of the haplotype A1-B8, especially for the benign epilepsy of childhood. The haplotype A1-B8 occured in none of the patients and B8 is expressed only by one patient. This shows the difficulties and the limitations of statistics when dealing with such small numbers.

Infantile Spasms

A study on HLA and infantile spasm was done by Howitz [7]. A sample of 21 patients showed no association with any HLA-A or -B antigen. Subdividing into those with symptomatic and idiopathic types made no difference.

Epilepsy with IgA Deficiency

In patients with epilepsy and IgA deficiency, HLA-A2 is significantly more frequent than in the control group or in epileptic patients without IgA deficiency (Table 4) [4, 13].

Table 4. HLA–A2 and epilepsy with IgA deficiency

Study	Patients		Control %+
	n	% +	
Fontana et al.	19	95	47
Shakir et al.	10	80	45

Photosensitivity

Westphal et al. [15] did not investigate the relationship between HLA and a special kind of epilepsy, but the relationship between HLA and a bioelectrical reaction, namely photosensitivity. Only photosensitive probands without seizures showed a significant association with HLA-Aw31 (Table 5). Therefore, these authors suggested that Aw31 could be a marker for a genetically determinated ability to prevent the manifestation of seizures.

Table 5. HLA–Aw 31 in photosensitive probands

With seizures		Without seizures		Control %+
n	% +	*n*	% +	
63	5	25	24	4

Family Studies

The only family study which looked at HLA and epilepsy was done by Scorza-Smeraldi et al. [12]. They investigated seven families in which one or more members were affected by primary generalized epilepsy (TCS, absences, juvenile myoclonic epilepsy) and/or displayed epileptic EEG patterns. In two families there was no segregation with the HLA locus, and in one family there may have been segregation with the HLA-A locus, but only if it was assumed that crossing over had occurred. (One cannot exclude this, because the parent was homozygous at the B and D locus.) The remaining four families showed a good agreement between HLA and disease inheritance. Nevertheless, the possibility that this happened by chance alone is very high, namely between 50% and 25%. Thus the seven families taken together do not provide evidence for linkage. Also, this is a heterogeneous group of epilepsies. An additional difficulty is, as in all genetic studies with epilepsy, that we do not know if an elderly person might have shown epileptic discharges at an early age.

Juvenile Myoclonic Epilepsy

We decided to look for an association between HLA and juvenile myoclonic epilepsy (JME) because JME is an ideal model for looking at genetic epilepsies. It is a specific and well-differentiated syndrome, there are no obvious exogenous factors that contribute to its etiology, and there is an increased incidence of the syndrome in family members [8]. In our sample, 75 unrelated patients with JME have now been typed for the A, B, C, and D locus by the bloodbank of the Klinikum Rudolf Virchow. Healthy blood donors typed in the same time period as the patients were used as controls. The phenotypic antigen frequencies were compared by the χ^2 test or Fisher's exact test. The p values were corrected by multiplying by the total number of antigens tested, after the Bonferoni inequality method.

After this correction no statistically significant association with antigens of the A, B, C or D locus was found. Also, there were no differences in the HLA antigen frequencies between patients who were and were not photosensitive or between those who had or did not have additional absence seizures.

Conclusions

No strong association with a specific antigen has been found in these investigations. On the contrary, results of the studies are highly inconsistent. A common problem in all studies of this kind is how to form homogeneous subgroups out of the diversity of the epilepsies. Subdividing the samples, means that the sample sizes are no longer large enough for any association to be detected.

Acknowledgement. This study was supported by grants from the Deutsche Forschungsgemeinschaft.

References

1. Eeg-Olofsson O, Säferenberg J, Wigertz A (1982) HLA and epilepsy: an investigation of different types of epilepsy in children and their families. Epilepsia 23:27–34
2. Eeg-Olofsson O, Osterland K, Guttmann RD, Andermann F, Olivier A, Janjua NA, Andermann E (1985) An immunological and genetic study of partial epilepsy. Can J Neurol Sci 12:210
3. Fichsel H, Kessler M (1980) Immunogenetics of 3/s-SW absence epilepsy: frequency of HLA antigens and haplotypes in patients and relatives. In: Canger R, Angeleri F, Penry JK (eds) Advances in epileptology: 11th epilepsy international symposium. Raven, New York
4. Fontana A, Joller H, Skvaril F, Grob P (1978) Immunological abnormalities and HLA antigen frequencies in IgA deficient patients with epilepsy. J Neurol Neurosurg Psychiatr 41:593–597
5. Gerstle de Pasquet E, Bolana C, Bonnevaux de Toma S, Perez-Campos H, Vila V, Alvarez I (1987) Immunogenetic studies in epilepsy. In: Wolf P, Dani M, Janz D, Dreifuss FE (eds) Advances in Epileptology, vol 16. Raven, New York, pp 599–602
6. Hafez M, Nagaty M, Saied E (1985) HLA antigens and idiopathic epilepsy. Epilepsia 26:15–18
7. Howitz P, Platz P (1978) Infantile spasms and HLA antigens. Arch Dis Child 53:680–682
8. Janz D, Durner M, Beck-Mannagetta G, Pantazis G (1989) Family studies on the genetics of juvenile myoclonic epilepsy (this volume)
9. Minev M, Martinova F, Belopitova (1987) On the association of the HLA-system with epilepsy in children. Epilepsia 28:74–76
10. Monoghan HP, O'Sullivan M, O'Donohoe NV (1982) HLA antigens and cryptogenic myoclonic epilepsy. Irish J Med Sci 151:188–189
11. Rivas ML (1983) Genetic analyses of petit mal epilepsy: I. Evaluation of HLA, blood groups, serum proteins and red cell enzymes. Epilepsia 24:115
12. Scorza-Smeraldi R, Cazzullo CL, Fabio G, Rugarli C, Smeraldi E, Canger R (1977) HLA antigens in primary generalized epilepsy. In: Penry JK (ed) Epilepsy. The 8th international symposium. Raven, New York, pp 317–323
13. Shakir RA, Behan PO, Dick H, Lambie DG (1978) Metabolism of immunoglobulin A, lymphocyte function and histocompatibility antigens in patients on anticonvulsants. J Neurol Neurosurg Psychiatr 41:307–311
14. Smeraldi E, Scorza-Smeraldi R, Cazzullo CL, Guareschi-Cazzullo A, Canger R (1976) A genetic approach to the Lennox-Gastaut-Syndrome by the histocompatibility complex (MHC) In: Janz D (ed) Epileptology. The 7th international symposium. Thieme, Stuttgart, pp 33–37
15. Westphal E, Gross-Selbeck G, Becker-Emner M, Doose H (1979) HLA-System, EEG und Epilepsie. In: Doose H, Gross-Selbeck G (eds) Epilepsie 1978. Thieme, Stuttgart, pp 221–225

Plasma Amino Acid and Genetic Studies in Epilepsy

N. A. Janjua [1], E. Andermann [1,2], O. Eeg-Olofsson [1], and B. Lemieux [3]

Historical Background

Historically, the interest in the study of biochemical constituents in the blood of patients with seizure disorders has existed since the beginning of this century. A number of studies during the early decades reported measurements of blood sugar, cholesterol, proteins, ammonia, uric acid, calcium, phosphorus, chlorides, etc. in epileptic patients (reviewed in [22]). None of these substances, however, were found to be consistently altered in association with epilepsy, and interest in the investigation of blood constituents in epileptic patients appeared to decline thereafter.

Measurements of free amino acids in the blood of epileptic patients were first carried out in the late 1950s. By the middle of the century, the concept of inborn errors of metabolism, as proposed by Garrod at the turn of the century, had become established and the search for metabolic defects in high-risk groups had gained impetus. As seizures were observed to be of common occurrence in inherited metabolic disorders, epilepsy qualified as a potential candidate for metabolic investigations. Hence, a few studies between 1959 and 1966 focused on amino acid investigations in the blood and/or urine of epileptic patients [12, 24, 40, 41, 47]. As a group, these studies seemed to indicate the presence of an abnormal aminoaciduria in epileptic patients, with or without accompanying changes in serum amino acid levels. The abnormal patterns of serum and urinary amino acid levels, however, did not resemble those associated with any of the inborn errors of metabolism known at the time. Furthermore, there were several inconsistencies among the studies, and the relationship of the changes in amino acid patterns to the etiology and mechanism of the seizures could not be defined.

For more than a decade following the early attempts at identifying an inborn error in amino acid metabolism in epilepsy, there seemed little interest in the measurement of amino acids in the blood or urine of epileptic patients. During this period, however, interest in the subject of heredity of epilepsy continued to grow as numerous clinical and EEG studies provided evidence to support the role of genetic factors in the etiology of epilepsy [2, 33, 35, 36, 38].

[1] Neurogenetics Unit, Montreal Neurological Institute, McGill University, 3801 University Street, Montreal, Quebec, Canada H3A 2B4.
[2] Centre for Human Genetics, McGill University, 1205 Ave. Dr. Penfield, Montreal, Quebec, Canada H3A 1B1.
[3] Department of Pediatrics, Centre Hospitalier Universitaire, Université de Sherbrooke, Sherbrooke, Quebec, Canada J1H 5N4.

Genetics of the Epilepsies
Beck-Mannagetta et al. (Eds.)

Recent Studies

During the past 15 years, a significant genetic contribution to the pathogenesis of epilepsy has been recognized [6, 7, 39, 43]. The precise nature of this contribution, however, still remains to be clarified. Over the years, different modes of inheritance have been postulated for different types of epilepsy or for specific epileptiform EEG patterns (reviewed in [43]). To date, however, no individual "epilepsy genes" or biochemical correlates for the clinically defined epilepsy traits have been identified.

Putative neurotransmitter amino acids are potential candidates for a role in the mechanism of epilepsy [11, 19, 34, 48]. Presently, a list of these amino acids includes glutamic acid and aspartic acid as excitatory and GABA, glycine, and possibly taurine as inhibitory neurotransmitters. Of these, glutamic acid and GABA have been more frequently implicated in the mechanism of epilepsy [19].

Most of the evidence implicating neurotransmitter amino acids in the mechanism of epilepsy is based on studies of experimental models of epilepsy. Only a few studies of human epilepsy have been carried out and results have been less conclusive. Large-scale neurochemical studies of neurotransmitter systems in humans are not feasible mainly due to difficulties in obtaining neural tissue from a large number of subjects. Neurochemical genetic studies of these systems in human families are virtually impossible due to the unavailability of neural tissue from unaffected family members of patients. Due to these limitations, attention is beginning to focus, once again, on nonneural tissues in studying the biochemical and genetic basis of epilepsy.

In 1980, van Gelder and co-workers [50] reported a significant increase in the plasma levels of glutamic acid and a significant decrease in aspartic acid and taurine in a group of patients with primary generalized corticoreticular (3/s spike-wave or absence) epilepsy and in their first-degree relatives. These findings could not be attributed to the effect of diet, anticonvulsants, or endocrine or maturational factors. The authors suggested that genetic factors were likely to play a role in determining the observed changes in the plasma levels of the three amino acids [50].

In two more recent studies as well [27, 28], a significant increase in plasma glutamic acid levels has been found in patients with primary generalized corticoreticular epilepsy and in their first-degree relatives, as well as in patients with focal epilepsy and in their first-degree relatives. Unlike the study by van Gelder et al. [50], however, a decrease in plasma aspartic acid and taurine levels was not observed by Janjua and co-workers [27, 28]. Moreover, in the latter studies, the mean plasma levels of aspartic acid were higher in both groups of patients and relatives as compared to controls, although the increase was not significant in all groups. The results of plasma amino acid investigations for glutamic acid, aspartic acid, and taurine for epileptic patients and for their first-degree relatives from the studies by van Gelder et al. and Janjua et al. are summarized in Fig. 1. It is important to note that none of the relatives in these studies had a clinical seizure disorder at the time of investigation or were receiving any anticonvulsant medication.

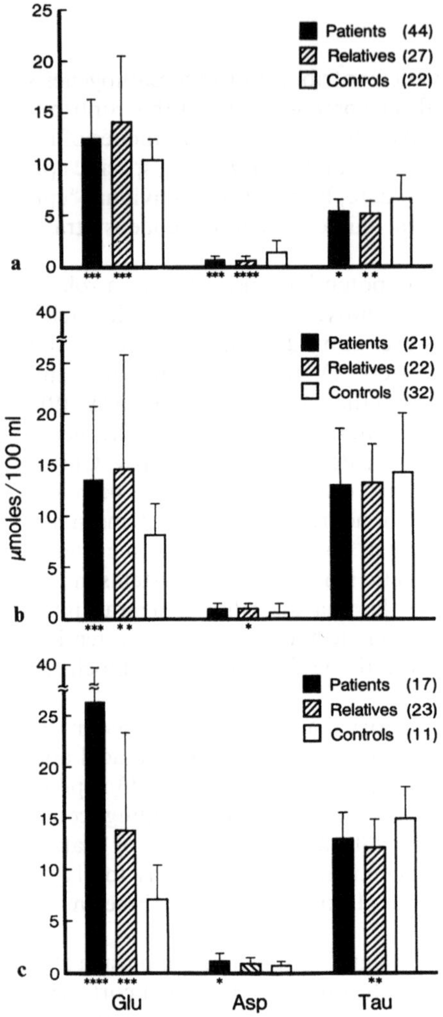

Fig. 1 a–c. Plasma glutamic acid (*Glu*), aspartic acid (*Asp*) and taurine (*Tau*) levels (mean ± SD) in epileptic patients and in their first-degree relatives. **a** Primary generalized corticoreticular epilepsy: from van Gelder et al. [50]. **b** Primary generalized corticoreticular epilepsy: from Janjua et al. [27]. **c** Focal epilepsy: from Janjua et al. [28]. Numbers in parentheses represent number of subjects in respective groups. Student *t*-test: $^{*}p<0.05$; $^{**}p<0.02$; $^{***}p<0.01$; $^{****}p<0.001$ as compared to controls

A significant increase in plasma glutamic acid levels in epileptic patients has also been observed in other studies in which family members were not investigated [26, 51]. With respect to aspartic acid and taurine, however, the results of these studies have, once again, been inconsistent. In the study by van Gelder et al. [51], the increase in glutamic acid was accompanied by unaltered aspartic acid and elevated taurine levels whereas Huxtable and co-workers [26] found elevated aspartic acid and unaltered taurine levels. These findings are summarized in Fig. 2. With respect to the type of epilepsy, the patients in these two studies comprised mixed groups (various seizure types and grand mal, respectively).

Among other plasma amino acid investigations in epileptic patients, unaltered levels of glutamic acid have also been reported [25, 42, 44]. In the studies by Plum

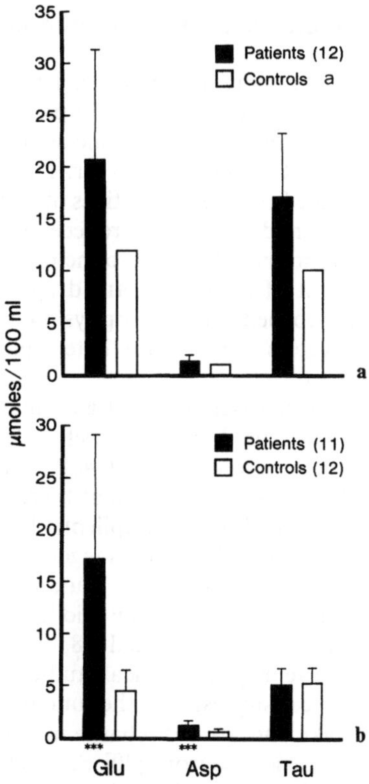

Fig. 2. a, b. Plasma glutamic acid (*Glu*), aspartic acid (*Asp*) and taurine (*Tau*) levels (mean ± SD) in epileptic patients. **a** Generalized and focal epilepsy: from van Gelder et al. [51]. **b** "Grand mal" epilepsy: from Huxtable et al. [26]. Numbers in parentheses represent number of subjects in respective groups. *a* Number of subjects not given. Bars represent maxima in the "normal expected range" from the literature. Student *t*-test: $***p<0.01$ as compared to controls

[44] and Haines et al. [25], this was accompanied by unchanged aspartic acid and taurine levels, whereas Monaco et al. [42] found elevated taurine levels. A significant increase in plasma taurine levels in epileptic patients has also been observed by Goodman et al. [23]. Plasma levels of glutamic acid and aspartic acid, however, were not measured in that study.

The reasons for the above mentioned discrepancies are not fully clear at present. At least some of these may be attributable to methodological differences, differences in the types of epilepsy studied, and the highly heterogeneous nature of the epileptic groups investigated [1, 25, 29]. These sources of variation may also explain, at least in part, the variation in findings with respect to other plasma amino acid changes in epilepsy. Significant alterations in the plasma levels of a number of amino acids other than glutamic acid, aspartic acid, and taurine, such as threonine, serine, methionine, isoleucine, leucine etc., have also been reported in epileptic patients (reviewed in [29]). These changes, however, have been observed much less frequently and have been far less consistent [29] than those discussed above.

Neurochemical, Neurophysiological, and Neurogenetic Perspectives

While many discrepancies between plasma amino acid investigations of human epilepsy carried out in the past 12 years remain to be resolved, the significant increase in plasma glutamic acid levels in epileptic patients appears to be the most consistent finding thus far. The fact that the increase in glutamic acid is observed in the first-degree relatives of epileptic patients as well, who neither have a clinical seizure disorder nor are receiving any anticonvulsants, suggests that this increase cannot be attributed to the neurophysiological phenomenon of seizures or to the effect of anticonvulsant drugs. Instead, the finding is compatible with several neurochemical, neurophysiological, and neurogenetic studies of epilepsy, and suggests a genetically determined role for glutamic acid in the etiology of epilepsy.

Decreased levels of glutamic acid have been reported in epileptogenic brain tissue from humans as well as from a variety of experimental models of epilepsy (for review see: [11, 29, 48]). Superfusion studies in cats and rats with cobalt-induced epilepsy show that there is a marked increase in the rate of release of glutamic acid from the epileptic focus [14, 15, 30, 31]. In light of this neurochemical evidence, it has been suggested that, in association with epilepsy, the capability of the CNS to retain glutamic acid may somehow be diminished. As a consequence, the glutamic acid levels in the extracellular space of the cortical neurons could become elevated [48, 49].

Neurophysiological studies in the penicillin model of generalized epilepsy in the cat suggest that the fundamental neurophysiological disturbance underlying spike and wave discharge may be a moderate diffuse increase in the excitability of cortical neurons [20]. Since glutamic acid has potent excitatory properties [32], its elevated levels in the extracellular space of the cortical neurons could be responsible for the hyperexcitability leading to the epileptic discharge [14, 15, 21, 49].

A number of recent genetic studies of epilepsy have suggested a multifactorial mode of inheritance involving interaction of both genetic and nongenetic factors [4, 5, 21]. A genetic predisposition or liability appears to be present in most types of epilepsy, including absence epilepsy with 3/s spike-wave EEG [38], focal epilepsy [2, 3] and febrile seizures [39]. The variety of clinical phenotypes is postulated to result from varying combinations of genetic and nongenetic factors [3, 21, 36].

The combined neurochemical, neurophysiological, and neurogenetic evidence presented above is compatible with the hypothesis that genetic predisposition to epilepsy may involve a gene-dependent biochemical derangement in the metabolism or transport of glutamic acid [21]. According to this hypothesis, such a defect when present in the cortical neurons will cause an increase in glutamic acid levels in the extracellular space, thereby leading to diffuse cortical neuronal hyperexcitability.

If it is assumed that a genetic defect in either the metabolism or the transport of glutamic acid underlies its excessive release from the epileptogenic brain tissue, then other tissues of the body can also be expected to have the *potential* to manifest that same defect. Results of plasma amino acid studies in epileptic patients and their relatives [27, 28, 50], in light of the preceding neurochemical, neurophysiological, and neurogenetic evidence, suggest that outside the CNS, the proposed genetic defect may be expressed in the form of elevated plasma glutamic acid levels. The mechanism of this glutamic acid increase in the plasma, however, as well as the specific nature of the defect in the brain remain unknown at the present time. The hypothesis that a common genetically determined aberration underlies glutamic acid changes in both the brain and the plasma assumes that: (a) the biochemical reaction(s) or the transport process(es), which may be the site of action of the gene(s) involved, are present both in the brain and in tissues outside the CNS; and (b) that these processes, both within and outside the CNS, are similar at the biochemical and molecular levels. These assumptions, of course, remain to be tested experimentally.

The proposed genetic defect in the metabolism or transport of glutamic acid in the CNS, which may be manifested in the plasma as well, is likely to represent one of the factors in the multifactorial etiology of epilepsy. The presence of this defect does not appear to be sufficient for the clinical manifestation of epilepsy since plasma glutamic acid levels are found to be elevated in the relatives of epileptic patients as well, even though these individuals do not have a clinical seizure disorder. Furthermore, patients with two types of epilepsy, which are distinct from the clinical and electroencephalographic points of view, namely primary generalized corticoreticular and focal epilepsy, show a similar increase in their plasma glutamic acid levels. Thus, elevation in glutamic acid in the plasma may be viewed as representing a genetic predisposing factor common to at least two types of epilepsy and perhaps to other types as well. However, additional factors, which may be both genetic and nongenetic, are necessary for the determination of the clinical and EEG phenotype.

Plasma Amino Acids as Biochemical Markers

A number of methodological difficulties and biases pertaining to the identification of affected individuals are encountered in the genetic and epidemiological studies of epilepsy [8–10, 35, 37]. Currently available diagnostic criteria, namely the occurrence of clinical seizures and of paroxysmal abnormalities in the electroencephalogram are not without pitfalls [8–10]. Due to these limitations, the need for a laboratory test that can reliably identify those individuals who have had or who might be at risk for having seizures has been emphasized [9]. If certain biochemical changes can be found to be associated with epilepsy, they can indeed serve as markers and hence facilitate the process of identification. To date, however, no reliable biochemical marker for epilepsy has been reported [17, 22, 29]. Significant alterations in plasma amino acid levels in epileptic patients and in their relatives may be conceived of as such markers, and thus may have significant implications for genetic and epidemiological investigations of epilepsy, where the aim of the investigator may be to identify individuals having a predisposition for seizures.

Thus far, however, it has not been possible to differentiate epileptic patients from controls with a high degree of accuracy using the plasma values of a single amino acid. Although many of the reported differences between epileptic patients and controls in the plasma values of indvidual amino acids have been highly significant, nevertheless, there has been overlap between the two populations. In the studies by van Gelder et al. [50] and by Janjua et al. [27, 28], for example, the increase in glutamic acid in epileptic patients and in their relatives is highly significant as compared to controls. However, it is not possible to distinguish all patients and relatives from all members of the control group on the basis of their plasma glutamic acid values. This may, once again, point toward the multifactorial etiology of epilepsy, suggesting that the increase in plasma glutamic acid levels may represent only one of the factors in the multifactorial etiology of epilepsy.

By using the plasma values of glutamic acid, in combination with values of some of the other amino acids, including aspartic acid and taurine, and employing discriminant analysis, it has been shown that patients with 3/s spike-wave epilepsy can be distinguished from controls with 100% accuracy [29]. However, since the significance of plasma amino acid changes in epilepsy, other than those involving glutamic acid, is less well-defined, the interpretation of these findings must await further studies. If significant changes in some of the other plasma amino acids are confirmed in association with epilepsy, then a biochemical profile based on plasma values of a group of amino acids may prove to be more useful than a single amino acid in differentiating epileptic patients from controls. This may also serve to further delineate the role of other amino acids such as aspartic acid and taurine, which have also been implicated in the mechanism of epilepsy [16, 34]. It is conceivable that amino acids other than glutamic acid may also be involved in, and thus may also contribute to, the multifactorial pathogenesis of epilepsy.

Concluding Remarks

Plasma amino acid studies in patients with well-defined types of epilepsy and in their families may offer a useful approach to the identification of a biochemical marker for genetic predisposition to epilepsy as well as to gain further insight into the basic mechanisms of the epilepsies. During the past 9 years, plasma amino acid investigations in patients with primary generalized corticoreticular epilepsy and in patients with focal epilepsy, as well as in the first-degree relatives of these subjects, have shown a significant elevation in plasma glutamic acid levels. The increase in glutamic acid is compatible with a number of previous neurochemical and neurophysiological studies, and appears to have a genetic basis. The precise nature of the genetic defect, however, remains speculative at present. Further studies involving determinations of enzyme activities in relevant metabolic pathways [46], transport mechanisms [45], receptors [18], and molecular genetic studies [13] are some of the approaches in the areas of contemporary biochemistry and molecular biology that could aid in the identification of the molecular basis underlying the amino acid changes in epilepsy.

Acknowledgements. This work was supported in part by the Johnson Foundation and the Savoy Foundation for Epilepsy. N.A.J. was the recipient of a postdoctoral fellowship from the Fonds de la Recherche en Santé du Québec. O.E.O. was a Visiting Scientist from the University of Linköping, Sweden, and was supported in part by the Swedish Medical Research Council (B83-19F-6407-01), and Margarethahemmet, Sweden. The secretarial help of Mary Huszthy was most appreciated.

References

1. Airaksinen EM, Oja SS, Marnela K-M, Leino E, Paakkonen L (1980) Effects of taurine treatment on epileptic patients. In: Battistin L, Hashim S, Lajtha A (eds) Neurochemistry and clinical neurology. Liss, New York, pp 157–166
2. Andermann E (1972) Focal epilepsy and related disorders: genetic, metabolic, and prognostic studies. Ph D Thesis, McGill University, Montreal
3. Andermann E (1980 a) Genetic aspects of epilepsy. In: Robb P (ed) Epilepsy updated: causes and treatment. Symposia Specialists, Miami, pp 11–24
4. Andermann E (1980 b) Multifactorial inheritance in the epilepsies. In: Canger R, Angeleri F, Penry JK (eds) Advances in epileptology: XIth Epilepsy International Symposium. Raven, New York, pp 297–309
5. Andermann E (1982) Multifactorial inheritance of generalized and focal epilepsy. In: Anderson VE, Hauser WA, Penry JK, Sing CF (eds) Genetic basis of the epilepsies. Raven, New York, pp 355–374
6. Andermann E (1985) Genetic aspects of the epilepsies. In: Sakai T, Tsuboi T (eds) Genetic aspects of human behaviour. Aino Hospital Foundation, Igaku-Shoin, Tokyo, pp 129–145
7. Anderson VE, Hauser WA, Penry JK, Sing CF (1982) Genetic basis of the epilepsies. Raven, New York
8. Annegers JF, Hauser WA, Elveback LR, Anderson VE, Kurland LT (1976) Seizure disorders in offspring of parents with a history of seizures – a maternal-paternal difference? Epilepsia 17:1–9
9. Baumann RJ, Marx MB, Leonidakis MG (1977) An estimate of the prevalence of epilepsy in a rural Appalachian population. Am J Epidemiol 106:42–52
10. Baumann RJ, Marx MB, Leonidakis MG (1978) Epilepsy in rural Kentucky: prevalence in a population of school age children. Epilepsia 19:75–80
11. Bradford HF (1975) On amino acid involvement in basic mechanisms of the epilepsies. In: Bradford HF, Marsden CD (eds) Biochemistry and neurology. Academic, London, pp 195–211
12. Choremis C, Kyriakides V, Karpouzas J (1959) Aminoaciduria in epilepsy. J Pediatr 55:593–601
13. Delgado-Escueta AV, White R, Greenberg DA, Treiman LJ (1986) Looking for epilepsy genes: Clinical and molecular genetic studies. In: Delgado-Escueta AV, Ward AA, Woodbury DM, Porter RJ (eds) Advances in neurology, vol 44. Basic mechanisms of the epilepsies: molecular and cellular approaches. Raven, New York, pp 77–95
14. Dodd PR, Bradford HF (1976) Release of amino acids from the maturing cobalt-induced epileptic focus. Brain Res 111:377–388
15. Dodd PR, Bradford HF, Abdul-Ghani AS, Cox DWG, Continho-Netto J (1980) Release of amino acids from chronic epileptic and sub-epileptic foci in vivo. Brain Res 193:505–517
16. Durelli L, Mutani R (1983) The current status of taurine in epilepsy. Clin Neuropharmacol 6(1):37–48
17. Eeg-Olofsson O, Janjua NA, Andermann E, Guttmann RD, Osterland K (1986) Immunological and genetic studies in primary generalized corticoreticular epilepsy. Acta Neurol Scand 74:425–431
18. Fagg GE (1985) L-Glutamate, excitatory amino acid receptors and brain function. Trends Neurosci 8(5):207–210
19. Fariello RG (1985) Biochemical approaches to seizure mechanisms: The GABA and glutamate systems. In: Porter RJ, Morselli PL (eds) The epilepsies. Butterworths, London, pp 1–19
20. Gloor P (1979) Generalized epilepsy with spike-and-wave discharge: a reinterpretation of its electrographic and clinical manifestations. Epilepsia 20:571–588

21. Gloor P, Metrakos J, Metrakos K, Andermann E, van Gelder N (1982) Neurophysiological, genetic and biochemical nature of the epileptic diathesis. In: Broughton RJ (ed) Henri Gastaut and the Marseilles School's contribution to the neurosciences (EEG suppl 35) Elsevier Biomedical, Amsterdam, pp 45–56
22. Goldstein H, McFarland RA (1940) The biochemistry of epilepsy: a review. Am J Psych 96:771–850
23. Goodman HO, Connolly BM, McLean W, Resnick M (1980) Taurine transport in epilepsy. Clin Chem 26:414–419
24. Gordon N, Wilson VK (1963) Abnormal amino-acid excretion in cerebral disease. Dev Med Child Neurol 5:586–592
25. Haines JL, Rich SS, Tsai MY, Anderson VE (1985) Altered amino acid levels in multiply affected sibships with seizures. Epilepsia 26(6):642–648
26. Huxtable RJ, Laird H, Lippincott SE, Walson P (1983) Epilepsy and the concentrations of plasma amino acids in humans. Neurochem Int 5(1):125–135
27. Janjua NA, Andermann E, Eeg-Olofsson O, Lemieux B, Giguère R (1989) Plasma amino acids in patients with primary generalized epilepsy and in their relatives. (Submitted to Ann Neurol)
28. Janjua NA, Eeg-Olofsson O, Andermann E, Lemieux B, Giguère R, Guttmann RD, Osterland K (1987) Plasma amino acid, immunological and genetic studies in patients treated surgically for focal epilepsy. In: Engel J Jr et al. (eds) Fundamental mechanisms of human brain function. Raven, New York, pp 267–278
29. Janjua NA, Metrakos JD, van Gelder NM (1982) Plasma amino acids in epilepsy. In: Anderson VE, Hauser WA, Penry JK, Sing CF (eds) Genetic basis of the epilepsies. Raven, New York, pp 181–197
30. Koyama I (1972) Amino acids in the cobalt-induced epileptogenic and non-epileptogenic cat's cortex. Can J Physiol Pharmacol 50:740–752
31. Koyama I, Jasper H (1977) Amino acid content of chronic undercut cortex of the cat in relation to electrical afterdischarge: comparison with cobalt epileptogenic lesions. Can J Physiol Pharmacol 55:523–536
32. Krnjevic K (1974) Chemical nature of synaptic transmission in vertebrates. Physiol Rev 54:418–540
33. Lennox WG, Lennox MA (1960) Epilepsy and related disorders, vol 2. Little, Brown, Boston, pp 532–574
34. Meldrum BS (1986) Drugs acting on amino acid neurotransmitters. In: Fahn S, Marsden CD, van Woert MH (eds) Advances in neurology, vol 43: Myoclonus. Raven, New York, pp 687–706
35. Metrakos JD, Metrakos K (1960) Genetics of convulsive disorders. I. Introduction, problems, methods, and base lines. Neurology 10(3):228–240
36. Metrakos JD, Metrakos K (1969) Genetic studies in clinical epilepsy. In: Jasper HH, Ward AA, Pope A (eds) Basic mechanisms of the epilepsies. Little, Brown, Boston, pp 700–708
37. Metrakos JD, Metrakos K (1970) Genetic factors in epilepsy. In: Niedermeyer E (ed) Modern problems of pharmacopsychiatry, vol 4: Epilepsy. Karger, Basel, pp 71–86
38. Metrakos K, Metrakos JD (1961) Genetics of convulsive disorders. II. Genetic and electroencephalographic studies in centrencephalic epilepsy. Neurology 11(6):474–483
39. Metrakos K, Metrakos JD (1974) Genetics of epilepsy. In: Vinken PJ, Bruyn GW (eds) Handbook of clinical neurology, vol 15. North-Holland, Amsterdam, pp 429–439
40. Millichap JG, Jones JD, Etheridge JE Jr (1966) The abnormal aminoaciduria in petit mal epilepsy. Neurology 16:569–572
41. Millichap JG, Ulrich JA (1962) Abnormal urinary excretion of amino acids in children with petit mal epilepsy: preliminary communication. Proc Mayo Clin 37:307–310
42. Monaco F, Mutani R, Durelli L, Delsedime M (1975) Free amino acids in serum of patients with epilepsy: significant increase in taurine. Epilepsia 16:245–249
43. Newmark ME, Penry JK (1980) Genetics of epilepsy: a review. Raven, New York
44. Plum CM (1975) Renal handling of free amino acids in normal adults, in patients with epilepsy, and in patients with Spielmeyer-Vogt-Batten disease. Dan Med Bull 22(5):194–201
45. Scriver CR, Rosenberg LE (1973) Amino acid metabolism and its disorders. Saunders, Philadelphia, pp 143–154

46. Sherwin A, Quesney F, Gauthier S, Olivier A, Robitaille Y, McQuaid P, Harvey C, van Gelder N (1984) Enzyme changes in actively spiking areas of human epileptic cerebral cortex. Neurology 34:927–933
47. Stemmermann MG (1965) Metabolic errors and seizures. Epilepsia 6:16–23
48. van Gelder NM (1978) Glutamic acid and epilepsy: the action of taurine. In: Barbeau A, Huxtable RJ (eds) Taurine and neurological disorders. Raven, New York, pp 387–402
49. van Gelder NM (1980) Glutamic acid metabolism and epilepsy (review). Jpn J NRA 6 (suppl):163–177
50. van Gelder NM, Janjua NA, Metrakos K, MacGibbon B, Metrakos JD (1980) Plasma amino acids in 3/sec spike-wave epilepsy. Neurochem Res 5(6):659–671
51. van Gelder NM, Sherwin AL, Sacks C, Andermann F (1975) Biochemical observations following administration of taurine to patients with epilepsy. Brain Res 94:297–306

Special Topics

Genetic Variability in Fetal Response to Anticonvulsants

D. LINDHOUT [1]

Introduction

Since the discovery of thalidomide embryopathy in 1961, many other drugs and chemicals have been recognized as potential teratogens. Observations during the last three decades have shown that thalidomide is still the strongest teratogen, causing malformations in 20%–50% of fetuses that are exposed during the critically sensitive embryonic period [20]. Only the retinoic acid congeners isotretinoin and etretinate and the obsolete trimethadiones induce severe anomalies in a similarly large proportion of exposed fetuses [13, 26, 31]. Most other teratogenic drugs are associated with malformations in a much smaller proportion of exposed fetuses. This is also the case with the anticonvulsant drugs phenytoin, phenobarbitone, primidone, valproate, and carbamazepine. The use of these drugs during the first trimester of pregnancy is associated with, on the average, a twofold risk of congenital malformation. High maternal serum levels of the parent drug seem to be of some significance [4, 12], but they cannot explain by themselves the occurrence of malformations because many unaffected infants were born after documented exposure to equally high maternal drug levels.

Genetically determined fetal and/or maternal susceptibility to specific teratogenic activity of anticonvulsant drugs may explain why only a small proportion of equally exposed fetuses react with malformation. This hypothesis is strongly supported by discordance for the fetal hydantoin syndrome in a pair of heteropaternal dizygotic twins of an epileptic mother using phenytoin throughout pregnancy [23]. This was also supported by a discordance for the thalidomide embryopathy that was observed in several pairs of dizygotic twins [20]; the genetically different twins were equally exposed and only one showed the specific teratogenic syndrome. In our own (unpublished) study of descendants of women treated for epilepsy we observed a nonrandom distribution of sibships without malformed infants and those with two or more affected infants, which supports the hypothesis of an interaction between the teratogenic drugs and one or more liable genes. In tests of pregnant animals, wide interspecies and interstrain differences in teratogen susceptibility is observed. This makes it often very difficult to predict the teratogenic potential of new drugs that are to be put on the market. Interindividual or interstrain differences in genetic susceptibility, however, may also have advantages. Identification and characterization of the teratogen susceptible genes in animals and humans may not only improve the accuracy of predicting, from ani-

[1] Department of Clinical Genetics, Erasmus University, P.O. Box 1738, 3000 DR Rotterdam, The Netherlands.

Genetics of the Epilepsies
Beck-Mannagetta et al. (Eds.)

Table 1. Maternal and fetal genetic factors in pharmacokinetics and drug response

Biological function	Genetic variables
Gastrointestinal resorption	Membrane transport Binding
Circulatory transport	Serum binding factors Serum converting factors
Metabolism	Hepatic enzymes Target tissue enzymes Metabolic activation Metabolic detoxification
Excretion	Renal Biliary Gastrointestinal
Pharmocodynamics	Receptors Other cellular targets
Maternal-fetal exchange	Placental transport Placental metabolism

mal findings, the human teratogenic potential of drugs but also provide us with better insight into the mechanisms of teratopathogenesis and with means to discriminate between teratogen-susceptible and -resistant persons and fetuses before therapy is begun. This will open the way to prevention of teratogenic side effects by rational drug choice based on genetic analysis before treatment, and to the development of newer drugs that are void of teratogenic activity even in susceptible individuals.

On the molecular-genetic level teratogen susceptibility is probably very heterogeneous. Table 1 summarizes possible sites where genetic variation may interfere with drug response, including adverse drug reactions. Most published experimental and human data concern genetic variability in microsomal drug metabolism. Animal experiments are currently the only source of data on the role of tissue receptors in teratogen susceptibility. Genetic factors interfering with gastrointestinal resorption, circulatory transport, and biliary and renal excretion have not been studied. Therefore, this review deals only with the genetics of drug metabolism although the potential significance of the other issues is recognized. The genetics of teratogen receptors will be reviewed elsewhere.

Genetic Variability in Drug Metabolism

All anticonvulsant drugs are subject to microsomal metabolism, which is under genetic control. In this system, lipophilic drugs are hydroxylated, glucuronated, or otherwise converted to substances that can be excreted through the kidneys or the biliary tract. Depending on the structure of the parent drug and the metabolic route, radical, usually short-lived intermediate metabolites are formed with potentially toxic effects on cellular functions. The epoxide-diol pathway is an ex-

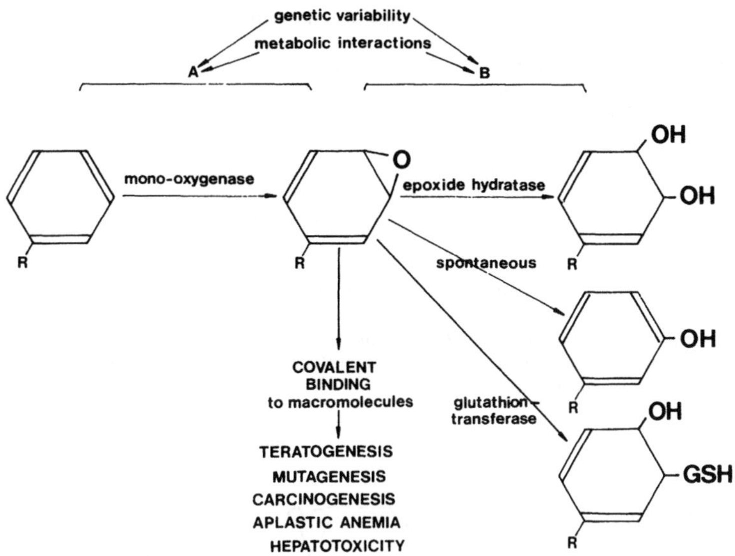

Fig. 1. The epoxide-diol pathway of drug metabolism. Metabolic activation as well as detoxification are susceptible to genetic variation or defects as well as metabolic autoinduction or interactions [18]

ample of such a metabolic route with production of potentially toxic metabolites (Fig. 1). The enzymatic processes that produce these intermediate metabolites are referred to as *metabolic activation*. The enzymes involved in the degradation of intermediate metabolites to less toxic or nontoxic compounds represent *metabolic detoxification*. One should notice that the same enzyme that activates a nontoxic substance into a toxic metabolite may inactivate the toxic metabolite of another compound into an inert metabolite. Thus, depending on the substrate, a drug-metabolizing enzyme can be involved in metabolic activation as well as in metabolic detoxification. A detoxified metabolite may undergo a subsequent conversion into a secondary or tertiary metabolite with strong toxic activity, as has been shown for benzo(*a*)pyrene where the dihydroxy-metabolite is subsequently converted into epoxide-diol-benzo(*a*)pyrene with a very strong toxicity [25].

An *imbalance* between metabolic activation and metabolic detoxification will modify the biological toxicity of the compound to which the organism is exposed. An absolute or relative increase in metabolic activation and/or a decrease in detoxification will render the organism more susceptible to the chemical agent, whereas a decrease in activation and/or an increase in detoxification will diminish the organism's susceptibility. This principle has been illustrated very well by animal experiments in which the teratogenesis of a specific compound was increased or decreased either through the modulation of metabolic activation/detoxification through pretreatment, or by the coadministration of enzyme inducers or inhibitors [19, 22, 29] (Table 2; Fig. 2). Support for this principle has also come from animal experiments showing strain differences in epoxide hydratase, which is associated with differences in teratogen susceptibility [7–9, 11]. Additionally, clini-

Table 2. Drug interactions and change in teratogenic risk

Subject	Teratogenic agent	Interacting agent	Teratogenic risk	References
Mice	Phenytoin	TCPO[a]	Increased	[19]
Humans	Carbamazepine or phenytoin	Phenobarbitone[b] + valproate[b] ± phenytoin[b]	Increased	[14]
Mice	Valproate	Phenobarbitone	Decreased	[22]
Humans	Valproate	Phenobarbitone	Decreased?	[16, 24]

[a] Trichloropropane oxide, a strong inhibitor of epoxide hydratase.
[b] Induction of monooxygenases by phenobarbitone ± phenytoin and inhibition of epoxide hydratase by valproate [3, 14].

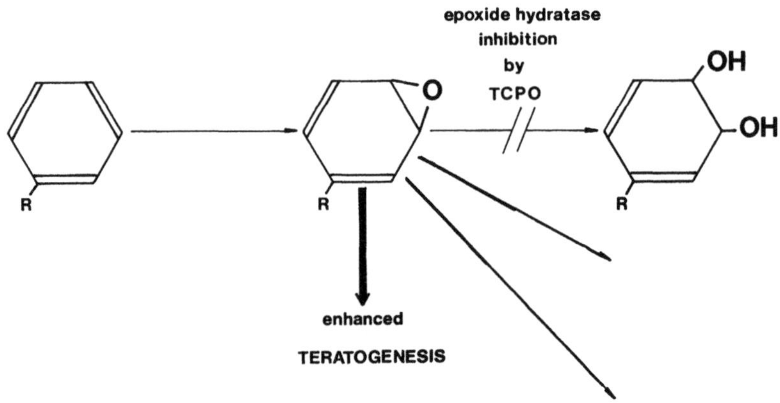

Fig. 2. TCPO inhibits epoxide hydratase with increased covalent binding of radiolabelled phenytoin to fetal tissues and induction of fetal malformations [19]

cal observation has shown an increased risk of congenital malformation with specific anticonvulsant drug combinations, characterized by an accumulation of epoxide metabolites [3, 14, 15, 17, 18] (Table 2; Fig. 3), and a decreased risk of VPA-induced spina bifida in valproate-phenobarbitone combination therapy, in which phenobarbitone accelerates detoxification of valproic acid VPA or one of its teratogenic metabolites [16, 24]. Variation in drug metabolism may have an effect on the teratogenic potential of drugs, and this implies that also *genetic* variation in human drug metabolism may play a significant role in individual susceptibility. Present knowledge of human pharmacogenetics shows that there is considerable variation between human individuals [1]. In our opinion, genetic variation in metabolic activation pathways, which usually has only a *proportional* increasing or decreasing effect on the production of intermediates, modulates the risk of side effects to exposed individuals which can only be measured by examining large exposed-patient groups or populations. On the other hand, a severe genetic defect in a detoxification pathway renders the individual organism very susceptible to

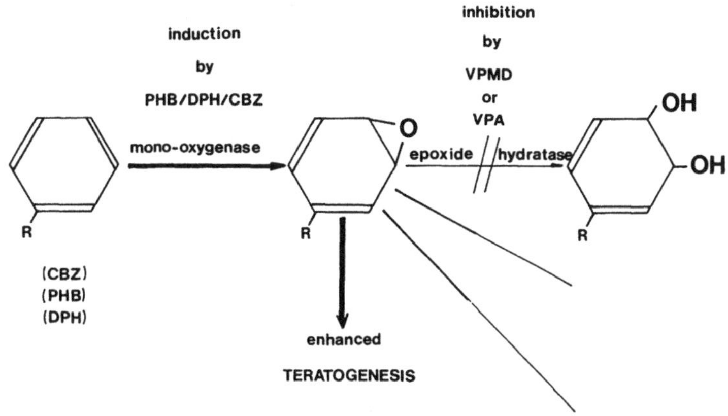

Fig. 3. The high risk of malformation after human fetal exposure to the combination of carbamazepine + phenobarbitone + valproate ± phenytoin may be explained by the accumulation of epoxide metabolites due to multiple drug interactions [3, 14]

the toxic intermediate that would normally be inactivated by the enzyme. A severe deficiency leads to a *disproportionately* strong accumulation of toxic intermediates and, subsequently to severe adverse drug reactions by the exposed individual (see Fig. 2). This could explain why a proportional increase in metabolic activation is usually associated with a variation in the relative risk of sporadic occurrences of, for instance, cancer and mutations, whereas a defect in metabolic detoxification may be associated predominantly with idiosyncratic drug reactions like aplastic anemia. hepatotoxicity, and fetal malformations.

Recently Strickler et al. demonstrated that peripheral lymphocytes isolated from malformed infants who had been exposed prenatally to phenytoin were more susceptible to the in vitro cytotoxic effects of intermediate phenytoin metabolites raised by microsomal enzymes that were added to the culture medium than lymphocytes from normal infants who had also been prenatally exposed to phenytoin [28]. The authors assumed a genetic deficiency in the detoxification of phenytoin intermediates to be present in lymphocytes of malformed phenytoin-exposed infants, possibly an epoxide-hydratase deficiency. Similarly, lymphocytes of patients with an idiosyncratic hepatotoxic reaction after halothane anesthesia were more susceptible to reactive phenytoin metabolites than lymphocytes of halothane-exposed patients without hepatoxemia [6]. The Strickler study deserves much attention because it is the first attempt to gain more insight into the genetics of individual teratogen susceptibility. Their positive findings will stimulate many of us to apply the pharmacogenetic approach – which has already been so successful in the study of mutagenesis, carcinogenesis, and experimental teratogenesis – also to the significant question of genetic susceptibility in human teratogenesis. The results of that study, however, deserve a critical comment. Not all exposed malformed infants had susceptible lymphocytes. Many of the infants whose lymphocytes were tested months or years after birth, and thus after exposure to phenytoin, had not been exposed to phenytoin exclusively, but also to other anticonvulsant drugs like phenobarbitone or primidone. These drugs strongly induce the cytochrome P-450-mediated monooxygenases, which include the metabolic activation pathway for phenytoin. Assuming there is a genetic defect in the detoxification of reactive phenytoin intermediates, induction of metabolic activation by comedication with phenobarbitone or primidone will increase the chance of an adverse drug reaction: Whereas a genetic defect in detoxification can only be clinically expressed when the fetus is exposed to the drug, this expression can be increased (or decreased) by comedication or other environmental factors interfering with drug metabolism. Strickler et al. might have found many more false-positive test results (more *normal,* phenytoin-exposed infants but with increased in vitro lymphocyte susceptibility) if the population examined had consisted only of infants that were prenatally exposed to phenytoin monotherapy.

Second, recent studies have shown that prenatal exposure to pharmacologically active compounds may permanently alter drug metabolism, even into adulthood. Adult rats that were perinatally exposed to maternally administered phenytoin showed persistent defects in hepatic monooxygenases. The changes consisted of depression in the velocity of aminopyrine-*N*-demethylase in 28-day-old rats, fetal sex-dependent changes in demethylase and hexobarbital hydroxylases in 4- to 5-month-old rats, and an impairment of phenobarbital induction in an otherwise normal phenytoin metabolism [27]. Administration of phenobarbital to mother rats during early lactation caused a long-term, perhaps permanent alteration of hepatic microsomal mixed-function oxidase activity (ethylmorphine-*N*-demethylase and aflatoxine-B1 adduct formation) in adult male offspring [21]. More or less similar experiments were done by others with phenobarbitone [2, 30] and benzo(*a*)pyrene [5] causing an increase and decrease, respectively, of hepatic monooxygenases in adulthood. This means that any specific defect in the metabolism of a compund to which an infant has been exposed prenatally might have been due to, and thus a secondary phenomenon of the prenatal exposure itself and not a primary genetic defect. One cannot, from the Strickler study, exclude that the prenatal exposure to phenytoin may have induced the malformations as well as a persistent deficiency in enzymatic detoxification in postnatal life, or that phenytoin-exposed nonmalformed infants with normal detoxification (resistent lymphocytes) may have been exposed to phenytoin in a way that was different from the malformed infants, e.g., to a lower dosage, lower serum levels, different or no comedications (phenobarbital, primidone), or other environmental factors.

Third, the end point of the lymphocyte susceptibility test was the ability or the loss of ability of the lymphocytes to exclude trypane blue or another vital stain. Therefore, the test outcome depends on the net exposure to the toxic metabolites, which is the result of many cellular factors including several different detoxification pathways. In particular, the test outcome may provide an estimate of the total detoxification (or all protecting or detoxifying cell factors) rather than a measurement of a single genetic defect.

Fourth, adult patients with an idiosyncratic drug reaction like aplastic anemia or hepatotoxemia showed a much stronger lymphocyte susceptibility to toxic drug metabolites than prenatally exposed malformed infants. The frequency of idiosyncratic drug reactions in exposed populations is of similar magnitude to that of homozygosity for an autosomal recessive metabolic disease in the general

Table 3. The search for fetal pharmacogenetic defects based on the diagnostic approach of hereditary metabolic diseases

Molecular level	Developmental stage	
	Prenatal	Postnatal
Metabolites (body fluids; intracellular)	Amniotic fluid (fetal serum)	Urine Serum (tissue)
Enzymes (activity, kinetics, inducibility, electrophoresis)	Chorionic villi Amniotic cells (fetal blood cells)	Blood cells Fibroblasts (tissue)
DNA (point mutations, deletions, RFLP linkage)	Chorionic villi Amniotic villi (fetal blood cells)	Blood leucocytes Fibroblasts
Biological assays (e. g. in vitro lymphocyte susceptibility)	Chorionic villi Amniotic cells (fetal blood cells)	Blood leucocytes (fibroblasts?)

population (1 in 10^4–10^5). The frequency of excess malformations due to fetal exposure to, for example phenytoin is about (0.7–2.0×10^2), which is similar to that of heterozygosity for a recessive disease in the general population. The fetal susceptibility to phenytoin teratogenesis may therefore be due to heterozygosity for a detoxification enzyme deficiency, for excample, epoxide hydratase, whereas the adult organism is less susceptible in the heterozygous state, and has to be homozygous for the gene defect to demonstrate idiosyncratic drug reactions. This hypothesis is in accordance with the observation of an intermediate in vitro response – as compared to the normal response of healthy controls and the strong response of patients with idiosyncratic drug reactions – by exposed malformed infants and at least one of their parents, as well as in the parents and some of the sibs of patients exhibiting idiosyncratic drug reactions. It is hardly conceivable, however, that this biological test can demonstrate heterozygosity with reasonable accuracy if we consider the common difficulties in heterozygosity testing for even single enzyme deficiencies by analysis of enzyme activity [10].

Defects in the structural gene for drug metabolizing enzymes, in regulatory genes, or in genes coding for receptors involved in enzyme induction usually remain unchanged, from conception throughout pre- and postnatal life. For this reason, the search for pharmacogenetic defects on the molecular DNA level is critically important. This represents the only level that can be examined in postnatal life and that still provides us with information on primary pharmacogenetic defects already present at conception, as opposed to secondary defects environmentally induced during embryonic or fetal development and persisting into infancy and adulthood. Characterization of such teratogen liability genes could provide a means for prevention by early and reliable detection of individuals at risk. The prospects for such a diagnostic approach are summarized in Table 3.

Summary

Several xenobiotics are subject to microsomal metabolism, which involves activation and detoxification pathways and the formation of intermediate metabolites. These metabolites may become toxic for example when there is covalent binding to cellular macromolecules like DNA, enzymes, or other proteins. They are also held responsible for the induction of idiosyncratic drug reactions in general, and hepatic failure, aplastic anemia, and birth defects in particular. Whether the organism is affected by one of these side effects depends not only on the type of drug or chemical and the sensitivity of the target (receptor variability), but also on the balance between metabolic activation and detoxification in the various tissues of the organism. Deficient detoxification, whether caused by inhibition due to metabolic interactions with coadministered drugs or chemicals, or caused by a genetic defect, may render the organism more susceptible to the occurrence of side effects.

A review is given of recent clinical and experimental studies including a discussion of the possible significance of their implications with respect to clinical antiepileptic drug use during pregnancy.

Acknowledgement. The author thanks Monique Steeman for her excellent secretarial assistence.

References

1. Agarwal DP, Goedde HW (1986) Pharmacogenetics and ecogenetics. Experientia 42:1148–1154
2. Bagley DM, Hayes JR (1986) Xenobiotic imprinting of the hepatic monooxygenase system. Effects of neonatal phenobarbital administration. Biochem Pharmacol 34:1007–1014
3. Chang S-L, Levy RH (1985) Inhibition of epoxidation of carbamazepine by valproic acid in the isolated perfused rat liver. J Pharmacokin Biopharmacol 13:453–466
4. Dansky LV, Andermann E, Rosenblatt D, Sherwin AL, Andermann F (1987) Anticonvulsant folate and pregnancy outcome: a prospective study. Ann Neurol 21:176–182
5. Faris RA, Campbell TC (1981) Exposure of newborn rats to pharmacologically active compounds may permanently alter carcinogen metabolism. Science 211:719–720
6. Farrell G, Prendergast D, Murray M (1985) Halothane hepatitis: detection of a constitutional susceptibility factor. N Engl J Med 313:1310–1314
7. Finnell RH, Chernoff GF (1984) Genetic background: the elusive component in the fetal hydantoin syndrome. Am J Med Genet 19:459–462
8. Finnell RH, Chernoff GF (1984) Variable patterns of malformation in the mouse fetal hydantoin syndrome. Am J Med Genet 19:463–471
9. Finnell RH, Chernoff GF (1987) Gene-teratogen interactions: an approach to understanding the metabolic basis of birth defects. In: Nau H, Scott J (eds) Pharmacokinetics in Teratogenesis, vol II. pp 97–112
10. Galjaard H (1980) Genetic metabolic diseases. Early diagnosis and prenatal analysis. Elsevier, Amsterdam
11. Hansen DK, Hodes ME (1982) Metabolism of phenytoin in teratogenesis susceptible and -resistant strains of mice. Drug Metab Dispos 11:21–24
12. Koch S, Jäger-Roman E, Rating D, Helge H (1983) Possible teratogenic effect of valproate during pregnancy. J Pediatr 103:1007
13. Lammer EJ, Chen DT, Hoar RM et al. (1985) Retinoic acid embryopathy. N Engl J Med 313:837–841

14. Lindhout D, Höppener RJEA, Meinardi H (1984) Teratogenicity of antiepileptic drug combinations with special emphasis on epoxidation (of carbamazepine). Epilepsia 25:77–83
15. Lindhout D, Verhoef A, Peters PWJ (1985) Teratogenicity of antiepileptic drug combinations as assessed by whole rat embryo culture. Teratology (abstracts) 32:27A–28A
16. Lindhout D, Schmidt D (1986) In-utero exposure to valproate and spina bifida. Lancet I:1392–1393
17. Lindhout D, Verhoef A, Peters PWJ (1986) Clinical and experimental teratogenicity of anticonvulsant drug combinations. Teratology (abstracts):33:7A
18. Lindhout D (1987) Teratogenicity of anticonvulsant drugs. Pediatr Update:129–147
19. Martz F, Failinger CIII, Blake DA (1977) Phenytoin teratogenesis: correlation between embryopathy effect and covalent binding of putative arene oxide metabolite in gestational tissue. Pharmacol Exp Therapeut 203:231–239
20. Mellin GW, Katzenstein M (1962) The saga of thalidomide: neuropathy to embryopathy, with case reports of congenital anomalies. N Engl J Med 267:1184–1244
21. Mitoma C, LeValley SE (1970) Effect on newborn rats of perinatal exposure to phenobarbital. Arch Int Pharmacodyn Ther 187:155–162
22. Nau H (1986) Valproic acid teratogenicity. Fundam Appl Toxicol 6:662–668
23. Phelan MC, Pellock JM, Nance WE (1982) Discordant expression of fetal hydantoin syndrome in heteropaternal dizygotic twins. N Engl J Med 307:99–101
24. Robert E, Rosa FW (1986) Human barbiturate teratology. Presentation at the workshop Pharmacokinetics in teratogenesis, Berlin
25. Robertson IGC, Jernström B (1986) The enzymatic conjugation of glutathion with Bay-region diol-epoxides of benzo(*a*)pyrene, benz(*a*)anthracene and chrysene. Carcinogenesis 7:1633–1636
26. Rosa FW, Wilk AL, Kelsey FO (1986) Teratogen update: vitamin A congeners. Teratology 33:355–364
27. Shapiro BH, Lech GM, Bardales RM (1986) Persistent defects in the hepatic monooxygenase system of adult rats exposed, perinatally, to maternally administered phenytoin. J Pharmacol Exp Ther 238:68–75
28. Strickler SM, Miller MA, Andermann E, Dansky LV, Seni M-H, Spielberg SP (1985) Genetic predisposition to phenytoin-induced birth defects. Lancet II:746–749
29. Wittkowski R, Verhoef A, Peters PWJ, Lindhout D, Nau H (1986) Pharmacokinetics of anticonvulsant drug combinations in pregnant rats. Teratology (abstracts) 33:61A
30. Yanai J (1979) Long term induction of microsomal drug oxidizing system in mice following prenatal exposure to barbiturate. Biochem Pharmacol 28:1429–1430
31. Zackai EH, Mellman WJ, Neiderer B et al. (1975) The fetal trimethadione syndrome. J Pediatr 87:280–284

Experimental Neurogenetics of the Epilepsies

J. L. NOEBELS [1]

Introduction

The inherited epilepsies are a heterogeneous group of neuronal diseases featuring abnormal paroxysmal cerebral discharges. Advances in their rational management depend upon interrelating two fundamental lines of clinical and basic research. The principal approach is descriptive, that is, to detect phenotypically similar clinical syndromes with informative pedigrees in order to isolate the shared genotypes and characterize their developmental expression in the brain. This search is now in progress for both man [8, 16] and animal [30], and may uncover useful chromosomal or biochemical markers to establish early diagnoses, provide new insights into the primary pathophysiologic mechanisms, and help clarify phenotypic variants of the disease arising from genomic diversity and epigenetic experience. A major expectation is that many of these genes, like the locus exemplified by Huntington's disease, which targets specific brain regions for programmed cell death [23], will illustrate an extraordinary selectivity for specific cell types sharing the inborn error. However, in the absence of neuronal markers for individual patterns of epileptiform discharges, the principal challenge centers on the difficulty of establishing a gene-linked primary lesion within the central nervous system and distinguishing it from the inevitable cascade of secondary pathological changes. As in other hereditary conditions, investigation of the nervous system in man is complicated above all by a requirement to defer molecular examination of the tissue until misleading terminal stages.

The second major neurogenetic approach toward epilepsy is experimental, and involves directly modifying the neurobiology of the epileptic nervous system to specifically prevent or correct patterns of abnormal cortical signaling. This general strategy is also beset with important limitations. Gene therapy that entails the incorporation of new DNA sequences into the germ line cannot be contemplated because recent studies in mammalian systems indicate that this process can introduce other deleterious mutations. Furthermore, unless the primary genetic error is nonneuronal, gene therapy in the somatic cell line cannot be accomplished a posteriori in a nondividing cell population. At present, the only realistic goal is to selectively alter expression of the existing genome, either by inducing or suppressing the transcription of genes, or by redirecting the posttranslational modification of their end products. The remarkable ability of the postmitotic neuron

[1] Department of Neurology, Section of Neurophysiology, Institute of Molecular Genetics, and The Blue Bird Developmental Neurogenetics Laboratory, Baylor College of Medicine, One Baylor Plaza, Houston, TX 77030, USA.

Genetics of the Epilepsies
Beck-Mannagetta et al. (Eds.)

to regulate membrane ion channel and receptor composition [7], neurite outgrowth [17], stabilization of synaptic contacts [4], and transmitter phenotype at central synapses [34] reaffirms the encouraging possibility that some diseases of paroxysmal neuronal membrane excitability, unlike the unremitting neurodegenerative disorders, may be reversible by compensatory modifications in specific networks of the mature central nervous system.

Defining "Epilepsy Genes"

Over 60 specific syndromes showing single-locus mendelian inheritance patterns have been associated with epilepsy [3, 24]. In some of these syndromes, however, seizures are not inevitable, and the pleomorphic effects of the gene may be significant. An instructive example is provided by recent molecular studies on one of these syndromes, Lesch-Nyhan syndrome, an *X*-linked disorder of purine metabolism, which results in a deficit of hypoxanthine phosphoribosyltransferase (HPRTase), hyperuricemia, and a complex congenital neurological disorder. Only half of the patients are subject to seizures [1]. Interestingly, the recombinant DNA-screening markers for HPRTase do not detect all affected patients [4], raising the liklihood of alternative mutant sequences. The ratio of those with a complete HPRTase deficiency to those with a seizure disorder who are correctly detected has not yet been ascertained. This disparity between the multiple clinical phenotypes and the spectral sensitivity of the molecular markers underscores the difficulty of analyzing even single-locus diseases in heterogenous populations.

The complex patterns of transmission observed in other families with epilepsy clearly indicate that multiple genetic loci exert important facilitatory or suppressant actions on the clinical appearance of epileptic phenotypes. Given the developmental plasticity and interdependence of the biophysical parameters controlling excitability and seizure threshold of cerebral cortex, the issue may frequently prove to be not whether but when (against what genetic background) a particular allele can be implicated as "epileptic." So far, in none of the inherited neurological syndromes with epilepsy has it yet been determined at the neurophysiological level exactly how the altered gene predisposes the brain toward seizure generation. This realization fully justifies the continuing efforts to formulate a more exact description of the membrane biophysics and the synaptic physiology underlying neuronal bursting and cortical EEG synchronization. Gene errors that fall short of generating a certain electroencephalographic sequence will not be recognized as epileptic phenotypes, even if the inciting cellular defect is largely the same. For the cellular neurophysiologist, then, the genetics of the epilepsies are the genetics of bursting neurons; in principle, the leading candidates for primary epilepsy genes are those encoding neuromodulatory mechanisms of repetitive firing as implicated by existing experimental models. Based on this broad definition, the list of determinants likely to play critical roles in inherited epilepsies includes the proteins involved in metabolism and release parameters of neurotransmitters and hormones, membrane receptor and ionchannel structural proteins, channel gating regulatory molecules, ion pumps and binding proteins, and the membrane surface adhesion molecules that determine cerebral organization and synaptic connectivity.

Identifying Excitability Genes

Defined in this manner, a representative sample of neuronal excitability genes has already been identified. In the "bottom-up" approach, using both reverse genetics and combined immunologic and recombinant DNA techniques allows isolation of either the mRNA or the DNA sequence and the construction of complementary probes. Table 1 lists some genes of potential interest identified in this manner. Using constructed probes for descriptive surveys, one might screen epileptic probands for mutations at the homologous loci. Experimentally, defined genetic models of epilepsy might be engineered by selectively mutating these genes in the normal animal. Although heteroduplex-induced site-directed mutagenesis of genes, using either sense [38] or antisense [15] sequences, can be demonstrated in transgenic culture systems, the method has not as yet been demonstrated in vivo.

The alternative strategy, a "top-down" approach, is based on an analysis of single locus mutations of inbred mouse strains in search of epileptic phenotypes [28]. As each is identified, the developmental expression of the lesion can be serially examined, one locus at a time, against the constant genetic background

Table 1. Cloned gene sequences relevant to inherited epilepsies

Category	Source	References
Ion channels		
Sodium	Rat	[27]
Receptors		
Acetylcholine (muscarinic)	Mouse	[25]
b Adrenoreceptor	Hamster	[10]
Neuropeptides		
Calcitonin	Rat	[2]
Cholecystokinin	Rat	[9]
Corticotrophin releasing factor	Sheep	[11]
Enkephalin	Human	[26]
Nerve growth factor	Mouse	[36]
Parathyroid hormone	Human	[39]
Prolactin	Human	[6]
Pro-opiomelanocortin	Human	[5]
Somatostatin	Human	[37]
Thyrotropin	Mouse	[12]
Vasoactive intestinal polypeptide	Human	[14]
Enzymes		
Dopamine-β-hydroxylase	Rat	[33]
Phenylalanine hydroxylase	Rat	[35]
Tyrosine hydroxylase	Rat	[18]
Protein kinase-camp dependent	Bovine	[19]

of the coisogenic strain, and compared directly with an unaffected littermate identical at virtually every other allele.

Single-Locus Mutants with Epilepsy

A simple strategy to find these mutations is to screen existing mapped neurological mutants in the mouse for behavioral or electrographic seizure activity. A partial listing of known epileptic mutants in the mouse is given in Table 2. The emerging results of this initial search reveal that genes for similar patterns of epilepsy are not rare, and are located on multiple chromosomes. This would be predicted not only on the basis of the number of experimentally identified pathologic mechanisms, e.g., differing ion channel or transmitter-receptor defects, but also by the observation that any one of these proteins typically depends upon several gene loci for normal expression. Molecular studies of the chromosomal arrangement of structural genes suggest that loci encoding subunits of single proteins are often dispersed. For example, four structural genes encoding the subunits of the nicotinic acetylcholine receptor have been localized to three chromosomes: the alpha subunit to chromosome 17, the beta subunit to chromosome 11, and the gamma and delta subunits to chromosome 1 in the mouse [13]. Other regulatory sites remain to be identified, and it is clear that mutations at any one of these sites might result in a compromised pattern of acetylcholine receptor expression.

Table 2. Single locus murine mutations with spontaneous epilepsy

Locus	(Symbol)	Chromosome	Mode	Pattern[a]
Lethargic	(lh)	2	rec	s/w arrest
Cribriform	(cri)	4	rec	convulsive
Leaner	(tgla)	8	rec	s/w arrest focal motor
Tottering	(tg)	8	rec	s/w arrest focal motor
Ducky	(du)	9	rec	s/w arrest focal motor
Staggerer	(sg)	9	rec	convulsive
Torpid	(td)	9	rec	convulsive
Dilute-lethal	(dl)	9	rec	convulsive
Mocha 2j	(mh2j)	10	rec	s/w arrest
Jittery	(ji)	10	rec	convulsive
Trembler	(Tr)	11	dom	convulsive
Wobbler-lethal	(wl)	14	rec	convulsive
Weaver	(wv)	16	rec	convulsive
Quaking	(qk)	17	rec	convulsive
Jumpy	(jp)	X	rec	convulsive

[a] Spike, or spike and wave EEG discharge with concomitant behavioral arrest; behavioral convulsion with postictal depression.

An Exemplary Mutation: The Tottering Mouse

The tottering mouse (*tg*, autosomal recessive, chromosome 8) displays an autosomal recessive neurological disease featuring ataxia, intermittant episodes of dystonic posturing and limb myoclonus, and frequent generalized bursts of 6–7 s spike and spike/wave cortical discharges [31]. The discharges last 1–10 s and are accompanied in every instance by a stereotyped arrest of behavior, an infrequent myoclonic jerk of the head or jaw, and vibrissal movements. Routine histopathology of the *tg* brain has not revealed any gross or microscopic findings when compared with the age-matched homozygous wild-type (+/+) littermate. Detailed studies of the central noradrenergic pathways have uncovered a striking and selective increase in both the level of noradrenaline (NE) and the number of noradrenergic terminals projecting to the forebrain, while the number of parent cell perikarya in the pontine nucleus locus ceruleus are unaffected [21]. Selective depletion of forebrain NE on the day of birth using a single intraperitoneal injection of 6-hydroxydopamine virtually eliminated the cortical discharges in the adult mouse [29]. Preliminary studies of *tg* brain show no alteration of alpha and beta adrenergic receptor populations [20], suggesting that the hyperinnervated target regions are not compensated by receptor down-regulation. Whether this apparent dysequilibrium represents a second defect within the catecholamine projection system, or the normal expression of receptor dynamics in a congenitally acquired lesion remains to be determined.

Summary

The primary goals of neurogenetic approaches to epilepsy are threefold: first, to identify major cerebral excitability loci and their modifiers, second, to map the regional and developmental expression of their end products, and third, to determine the reversibility of both the primary cellular lesions and their secondary actions on brain development. Analysis of mutations causing seizures in mice offer an important opportunity to extend the classification of inherited epilepsies to the level of membrane diseases, and to formulate more selective antiepileptic agents and a specific developmental timetable for initiating therapy.

The author is supported by NIH grant NS 11535-12, a Basil O'Connor award (March of Dimes/Birth Defects Foundation, the Pew Foundation) and the Bluebird Circle Foundation.

References

1. Adams RD, Lyon G (1982) Neurology of hereditary metabolic diseases of children. McGraw-Hill, New York
2. Amara SG, Jonas V, Rosenfield BA, Ong ES, Evans RM (1982) Alternative RNA processing in calcitonin gene expression generates mRNAs encoding different polypeptide products. Nature 298:240–244
3. Anderson VE, Hauser WA, Rich S (1986) Genetic heterogeneity in the epilepsies. Adv Neurol 44:59–76

4. Changeux JP, Danchin A (1976) Selective stabilization of developing synapses as a mechanism for the specification of neuronal networks. Nature 264:705–712
5. Cochet M, Chang ACA, Cohen SN (1982) Characterization of the structural gene and putative 5′ regulatory sequences for human proopiomelanocortin. Nature 297:335–339
6. Cooke HE, Baxter JD (1982) Structural analysis of the prolactin gene suggests a separate origin for its 5′ end. Nature 297:602–606
7. Cotman CW, Nieto-Sampedro M (1984) Cell biology of synaptic plasticity. Science 225:1287–1294
8. Delgado-Escueta A, White R, Greenburg D, Treiman L (1986) Looking for epilepsy genes. Adv Neurol 44:77–96
9. Deschenes R, Lorenz L, Haun R, Roos BA, Collier KC, Dixon JE (1984) Cloning and characterization of mRNA encording a rat cholecystokinin. PNAS 81:726–730
10. Dixon RAF et al. (1986) Cloning of the gene and cDNA for mammalian B-adrenergic receptor and homology with rhodopsin. Nature 321:75–79
11. Furutani Y, Morimoto Y, Shibahara S, Noda M, Takahashi H, Hirose T, Asai M, Mayama S, Miyata T, Numa S (1983) Cloning and sequence analysis of cDNA for ovine corticotropin releasing factor precursor. Nature 301:537–540
12. Gurr JA, Catterall JF, Kourides IA (1983) Cloning of cDNA encoding the pre B subunit of mouse thyrotropin. PNAS 80:2122–2126
13. Heidmann O, Buonanno A, Geoffroy B, Robert B, Guenet JL, Merlie JP, Changeux JP (1986) Chromosomal localization of muscle nicotinic acetylcholine receptor genes in the mouse. Science 234:866–868
14. Itoh N, Obata L, Yanaihar N, Okamoto H (1983) Human preprovasoactive intestinal polypeptide contains a novel PHI-27-like peptide PHM-27. Nature 304:547–549
15. Izant JG, Weintraub H (1984) Inhibition of thymidine kinase gene expression by anti-sense RNA: a molecular approach to genetic analysis. Cell 36:1007–1015
16. Janz D (chapter 7 in this book)
17. Korsching S (1986) The role of nerve growth factor in the CNS. Trends Neurosci 9:570–573
18. Lamouroux A, Bignet NF, Samolyk D, Privat A, Salomon JC, Pujol JF, Mallet J (1982) Identification of cDNA clones coding for rat tyrosine hydroxylase antigen. PNAS 79:3881–3885
19. Lee DC, Carmichael DF, Krebs EG, McKnight S (1983) Isolation of a cDNA clone for the type 1 regulatory subunit of bovine cAMP-dependent protein kinase. PNAS 80:3208–3212
20. Levitt P, Lau C, Pylypiw A, Ross LL (1984) Central adrenergic receptors in the inherited noradrenergic hyperinnervated mutant mouse tottering. Brain Res 418:174–177
21. Levitt P, Noebels JL (1981) Mutant mouse tottering: selective increase of locus coeruleus axons in a defined single locus mutation. PNAS 78:4630–4634
22. Liles WC, Taylor S, Finnell R, Lai H, Nathanson NM (1986) Decreased muscarinic acetylcholine receptor number in the central nervous system of the tottering mouse. J Neurochem 46:977–982
23. Martin JB (1982) Huntingtons disease: genetically determined cell death in the mature human nervous system. In: Schmitt FO, Bird SJ, Bloom FE (eds) Molecular genetic neuroscience. Raven, New York
24. McKusick VA (1983) Mendelian inheritance in man, 6th edn. Johns Hopkins University Press, Baltimore
25. Merlie JP, Sebbane R, Gardner S, Lindstrom J (1983) cDNA clone for the subunit of the acetylcholine receptor from the mouse muscle cell line BC3H-1. PNAS 80:3845–3849
26. Noda M, Teranishi Y, Takahashi H, Toyasato M, Notake M, Nakanishi S, Numa S (1982) Isolation and structural organization of the human preproenkephalin gene. Nature 297:431–434
27. Noda M, Ikeda T, Kayano T, Suzuki H, Takeshima H, Kurasaki M, Takahashi H, Numa S (1986) Existence of distinct sodium channel messenger RNAs in rat brain. Nature 320:188–192
28. Noebels JL (1979) Analysis of inherited epilepsy using single locus mutations in mice. Fed Proc 38:2405–2410

29. Noebels JL (1984) A single gene error of noradrenergic axon growth synchronizes central neurons. Nature 310:409–411
30. Noebels JL (1986) Mutational analysis of inherited epilepsies. Adv Neurol 44:97–114
31. Noebels JL, Sidman RL (1979) Inherited epilepsy: spike wave and focal motor seizures in the mutant mouse tottering. Science 204:1334–1336
32. Noebels JL, Beal MF, Martin JB, Holets-Whittemore VR, Hokfelt T (1985) Neuropeptide Y levels in a gene mutation causing central noradrenergic hyperinnervation. Neurosci Abstr 15:140
33. O'Malley KL, Mauron A, Rase J, Barchas JD, Kedes L (1983) Genes for catecholamine biosynthesis: cloning by expression and identification of the cDNA for rat dopamine-B-hydroxylase. PNAS 80:2161–2165
34. Park JK, Joh TH, Ebner FF (1986) Tyrosine hydroxylase is expressed by neocortical neurons after transplantation. PNAS 83:7495–7498
35. Robson KJH, Chadra T, MacGillivray RTA, Woo SLC (1982) Polysome immunoprecipitation of phenylalanine hydroxylase mRNA from rat liver and cloning of its cDNA. PNAS 79:4701–4705
36. Scott J, Selby M, Urdea M, Quiroga M, Bell GI, Rutter WJ (1983) Isolation and nucleotide sequence of a cDNA encoding the precursor of mouse nerve growth factor. Nature 302:538–540
37. Shen LP, Pictet RL, Rutter WJ (1982) Human somatostatin I sequence of the cDNA. PNAS 79:4575–4579
38. Thomas KR, Capecchi MR (1986) Introduction of homologous DNA sequences into mammalian cells induces mutations in the cognate gene. Nature 324:34–38
39. Vasicek TJ, McDevitt BE, Freeman MW, Fennick BJ, Hendy GN, Potts JT, Rich A, Kronenberg HM (1983) Nucleotide sequence of human parathyroid hormone gene. PNAS 80:2127–2131
40. Willow M, Taylor SM, Catterall WA, Finnell RH (1986) Down regulation of sodium channels in nerve terminals of spontaneously epileptic mice. Cell Molec Neurobiol 6:213–220
41. Yang TP, Patel P, Chinault A, Stout J, Jackson L, Hildebrand B, Caskey CT (1984) Molecular evidence for new mutation at the hprt locus in Lesch Nyhan patients. Nature 310:412–414

Perspectives: Clues in Mapping Epilepsy Genes

A. V. DELGADO-ESCUETA [1], D. A. GREENBERG [2], and L. TREIMAN [1]

Introduction

Soon it will be possible to practice medicine at a molecular level and identify gene products by mapping genes for a growing number of diseases, including the epilepsies. The chromosomal locations of about 900 structural genes are now known, representing less than 2% of the total 50000 genes estimated for man (McKusick [50]). In addition, 500 anonymous DNA segments have been mapped to specific human chromosomes and many of these human genes have sequence variations, making them useful linkage markers.

This article covers two main topics. First, genetic methodologies currently used to explore the genetics of epilepsy will be discussed: these include not only segregation analysis and classical linkage studies but also recombinant DNA technology for screening genes that may cause the disease. Second, juvenile myoclonic epilepsy and an early childhood epilepsy syndrome, two forms of idiopathic generalized epilepsy, will be discussed, proofs for a strong genetic component presented, and clues to their chromosomal sites discussed.

Heterogeneity of Epilepsies

One overriding fact must be considered when addressing the question of the genetics of epilepsy, namely that the various epilepsies are heterogenous. As such, there are "genetic" forms and "non-genetic" (i.e., environmental) forms that appear clinically identical. There are also a variety of genetic forms that appear identical clinically. Such diversity could be the result of different genetic loci (that is, different locations on the human genome) or different alleles at the same locus. In addition, there are undoubtedly different modes of inheritance for different epilepsies. Further confusing the issue is the question of "genetic susceptibility" to epilepsy that may underlie the development of partial epilepsy after focal brain damage in natal and postnatal head injury, infections, and neoplasms. In planning genetic studies, it is generally asked: What proof is there that epilepsy genes exist? And which forms of epilepsy would be best suited for genetic linkage studies?

[1] Reed Neurological Research Center, UCLA School of Medicine, 710 Westwood Plaza, Los Angeles, CA 90024, USA.
[2] Southwest Regional VA Epilepsy Center, Neurology Service, Wadsworth VA Medical Center, Los Angeles. Current address: Department of Psychiatry, Mt. Sinai Medical Center, 1 Gustave Levy Place, New York, NY 10029, USA.

Genetics of the Epilepsies
Beck-Mannagetta et al. (Eds.)

The best current evidence for the existence of epilepsy mutant genes in the human population comes from family studies which look for familial clustering in specific forms of epilepsy. Twin studies demonstrate a major genetic factor in idiopathic generalized epilepsies. The overall concordance rate for epilepsy reported in six major twin studies was 60.2% for monozygotic pairs and 13.2% for dizygotic pairs (Tsuboi [83]). If twin studies are confined to absence seizures and generalized tonic-clonic convulsions and pairs are examined at the peak age of phenotypic expressions (6–18 years), the concordance rate is 100%. Lennox and Lennox [45] noted that when epilepsies without organic brain lesions were identified, concordance was 70.2% (33 out of 47) for monozygotic twins and 5.6% (3 out of 54) for dizygotic pairs. When they confined their analysis to 30 twin pairs with spike and wave traits in the EEG, concordance was 74% for the spike and wave trait in monozygotic and 27% for dizygotic twins. Gedda and Tatarelli [24] identified 45 pairs of twins with primarily generalized seizures and reported concordance rates of 94.7% in 19 monozygotic twins and 15.4% in 26 dizygotic twins.

The partial epilepsies are usually thought of as acquired and caused by specific structural cerebral lesions, the pattern of seizures being determined by the area of cortical involvement. While some studies have demonstrated a greater incidence of epilepsies among first-degree relatives of patients with partial seizures than in relatives of control patients, results are not unequivocal. Rimoin and Metrakos [70] studied the incidence of seizures in families of children with infantile hemiplegia. Seizures occurred more frequently in families of children who had both hemiplegia and seizures than in control families. In comparison with control families, however, the incidence of seizures was *lower* in the families of children with hemiplegia but no seizures. Obviously, the question of susceptibility to epilepsy after head trauma is extremely difficult to investigate. Once we have clarified the genetic picture in the genetic epilepsies, we will have much better tools with which to investigate genetic sensitivity to trauma that may lead to epilepsy.

Linking Chromosomal Markers to Epilepsies

Linkage analysis uses standard genetic markers (Table 1), anonymous DNA markers called restriction fragment length polymorphisms (RFLP's; Botstein et al. [6]), and candidate gene markers (White [93]; Caskey and White [7]), to find the chromosomal location of the disease gene (Haldane and Smith [28]; Mohr [52]; Morton [54]; Conneally and Rivas [9]). The basis of the method is to test for the cosegregation, *within families*, of the markers with the disease. It is important that linkage be distinguished from association. In association, a *specific allele* of some marker locus, such as HLA-B27, is found more frequently in people affected with the disease, such as ankylosing spondylitis, than is found in the general population. In linkage analysis, a specific marker allele and the disease are *not* found together more frequently in the population of affected individuals than in the general population. What is important in linkage analysis is that, *within families,* some marker allele be found together with the disease more often than would be expected on the basis of an assumption of independent segregation of loci.

Table 1. Polymorphic gene markers currently evaluated at the UCLA biochemical genetics laboratory and their assigned chromosome locations[a] (chromosome assignments from Shows et al. [77]

Red blood cell Antigens	Chromosome assignment	Red blood cell enzymes	Chromosome assignment	Serum proteins	Chromosome assignment
ABO	9	6-Phosphogluconate dehydrogenase	1	Haptoglobin	16
Lewis	19	Adenylate kinase$_1$	9	Transferrin	?
Rh	1	Adenosine deaminase	20	Pseudocholinesterase	?
MNSs	4	Acid phosphatase	2	Complement C3	19
Duffy	1	Glutamic pyruvate transaminase	8 (?)	Gc component	4
Lutheran	19	Phosphoglucomutase$_1$	1	Alpha$_1$-antitrypsin	14
Kell	?	Galactose$_1$-phosphate uridyl transferase	9	Serum amylase	1
Kidd	2 (?)	Esterase D	13	Gm	14
P	6 (?)	Peptidase A	18	Properdin factor B (BF)	6
Xga	X	Glucose-6-phosphate dehydrogenase	X		
		Phosphoglycolate phosphatase	16		

[a] ? indicates chromosome unknown or assignment provisional.

Unlike testing of candidate genes, linkage analysis can be carried out without any previous notion of where the disease locus is found on the human genome. Indeed, its purpose is to locate the disease locus relative to a genetic marker whose chromosomal site is already known. Such chromosomal markers may consist of phenotypic blood groups, proteins, and enzymes (Table 1), anonymous DNA markers (RFLPs), and candidate gene markers (see Table 2).

It has been estimated that an evenly spaced set of less than 100 highly polymorphic genetic markers would completely cover the human genome (Shows et al. [76]). The significance of this estimate is that such a set of markers would reliably detect genetic linkage with any unknown genetic disease locus (such as a locus for juvenile myoclonic epilepsy), not only establishing its map location but also confirming the primary role of a genetic component in the disease process.

Linkage analysis also estimates the chromosomal map distances between the marker gene and the epilepsy gene. These distances are expressed in morgans and centimorgans; one centimorgan map unit (cM), or approximately 10^6 base pairs of DNA, means 1% recombination. At a distance of 1.0 cM, two alleles which are on the same chromosome in the parent will be inherited together 99% of the time. With increasing distance there is more likelihood that the two alleles will be inherited on different chromosomes. Thus, linkage in multiplex epilepsy families will be detected with confidence if the locus for the marker and the locus for epilepsy are inherited together 90% of the time, or at a distance of 10 cM (Conneally and Rivas [9]).

The criterion for the existence or not of linkage between two loci is the "lod" (log of the odds) score. This expresses the odds of the hypothesis in favor of linkage against the hypothesis of no linkage. A lod score of 1 means 10:1 odds in favor of linkage over no linkage, while a lod score of 5 would mean 100000:1 in favor of linkage. Generally, a score of 3 (1000:1) is considered to demonstrate linkage if the mode of inheritance is known, while a score of −2 (1:100 in favor of no linkage) is considered proof that no linkage exists if the mode of inheritance is known (Mohr [52]; Morton [54]).

When linkage analysis is undertaken, a mode of inheritance must be specified. However, it is possible to carry it out without knowledge of the mode of inheritance by performing the analysis assuming different modes of inheritance. Hodge et al. [32], for example, have shown that linkage analysis results for their data remained reasonably stable under the assumption of different modes of inheritance. Morton [54] and others (e.g. Ott [59]) have attempted to combine linkage analysis and segregation analysis into complementary methods, rather than having linkage analysis dependent on segregation analysis. There are now, also, statistically based methods that can detect heterogeneity in a linkage data set. This is of utmost importance because linkage analysis operates on the assumption that only one disease or one form of epilepsy is being studied. If a biological way can be developed of differentiating the various forms of epilepsies, these methods can provide supporting evidence that heterogeneity exists.

Linkage with Standard Genetic Markers and RFLPs

What makes linkage analysis difficult in practice is that tissue samples from entire families must be collected and the phenotypes of family members at marker loci determined before the analysis can be carried out. Moreover, the location of the disease gene is relative to a known marker. If one has no idea where the disease gene is located, which is usually the case, then many marker loci must be examined. Fortunately, the number of genetic markers that can be used in linkage analysis has expanded at least tenfold because of the emergence of RFLP (Botstein et al. [6]). RFLP methods involve cutting the whole DNA into fragments using restriction enzymes. Restriction enzymes are bacterial enzymes that cut the DNA at a specific sequence of bases (ATTAG, for example). These cut points, as they are called, are randomly distributed throughout the genome, and can be considered markers. A piece of DNA from a specific part of the genome that is 1000 bases long in one person may be 5000 bases long in another, because the second person lacks a cut point at that location (hence the word "length" in "restriction fragment length polymorphism"). These fragments of DNA are then separated by size using agarose gel electrophoresis (Southern [79]). In the final step the blot is treated with a DNA probe (a radioactively labeled probe) and then anneals to its complementary DNA from the genome. The location on the blot where it anneals to its complementary DNA will be determined by the size of the fragment of genomic DNA that was produced with the restriction enzyme. One of the things that makes this approach so potentially useful is that, since there are hundreds of restriction enzymes, the number of potential markers is enormous.

A polymorphic locus is therefore generally defined by two factors: the probe which defines the genetic locus, and application of a restriction enzyme or enzymes to a set of individuals to provide fragments for a population sample to define alleles. In developing a strategy for revealing RFLPs one must consider the number and nature of the individuals afflicted with epilepsies, the enzymes, the probes used in screening, and how polymorphic an RFLP is (White [93]).

Confirming inheritance and measuring recombination distances can be carried out in kindreds with juvenile myoclonic epilepsy. Skolnick and White [78] suggest that screening at least nine individuals in a kindred is adequate: although a large proportion of rare variants and a few of the marginal polymorphisms will be missed, the majority of the most useful polymorphisms will be captured.

The selection of enzymes is an important factor in the design of a screen for DNA polymorphisms. There are essentially two varieties of DNA polymorphism: those that arise from base-pair substitution polymorphism and those that arise from small deletions or insertions in chromosome rearrangements. Base-pair substitutions can alter a restriction enzyme recognition site, while deletions or insertions of large sequences alter fragment patterns without altering recognition sites.

The screen for base-pair substitution polymorphisms is enhanced by any enzyme that detects restriction sites different from those already screened. Each screen detects two restriction sites, one extending past each end of the sequence which hybridizes with the probe. In general screening, efficiency for base-pair substitution is increased with long probes and enzymes that produce short fragments. Skolnick and White [78] use *MspI* which recognizes CCGG and *TaQI* which recognizes TCGA. The screen is inefficient for RFLPs of less than 200 base pairs since they are not revealed in hybridization experiments. Base-pair substitution polymorphisms are relatively abundant (in about 20% of single-copy probes), whereas detectable insertion-deletions have been found in only one of approximately 50 probes screened. An enzyme such as *KpnI* is used to screen for deletions.

Screening with Candidate Gene Markers

In the epilepsies, where two decades of fruitful research have implicated several proteins as important in the expression of the disease, the approach of choice is

Table 2. Candidate gene markers for epilepsy

Proteins hypothesized to have a role in epileptogenesis	Available monoclonal antibodies	Unique DNA sequences	Chromosome
$Na^+K^+ATPase$	Albers et al. (1984)	Sheep kidney –	?
Alpha subunit	Siegel et al. (1985)	Shull et al. (1985)	
$Alpha^+$ (not done)	Fambrough et al.	Torpedo electric organ –	
Beta subunit (not done)	(1985)	Kawakami et al. (1985)	
$Ca^{2+}ATPase$	MacLennan et al. (1985)	MacLennan et al. (1985)	?
Na^+ channel protein	Noda et al. (1984)	Noda et al. (1984)	?
Ca^{2+} calmodulin kinase	DeLorenzo (1985)	In development (1986) Wasterlain	?
Protein kinase C	Ullrich et al. (1984)	Parker et al. (1986)	?
Cyclic AMP-dependent protein kinase	Ullrich et al. (1984)	Parker et al. (1986)	?
GABA-benzodiazepine receptor	Olsen et al. (1985)	In development, Olsen	?
Glutamic acid decarboxylase	Salveterra et al. (1983) Kopin et al. (1982)	Tobin (1986)	2

probably to search for polymorphisms for specified cloned genes of proteins shown to be abnormal in epilepsies of humans and experimental animals (candidate gene markers; White [93]). In the epilepsies, prior reasons exist for suspecting the genes for the GABA receptor (Olsen et al. [58]), the Na^+K^+ pump (Towers [82]; Grisar et al. [25]; Rapport et al. [68]), the gating proteins for the Na^+ channel, K^+ channel, and Ca^{2+} channel (Narahashi [55]), and membrane enzymes involved in conduction-secretion coupling (DeLorenzo [14]; Table 2). One can look for linkage between the DNA of cloned proteins and the disease segregating in a pedigree. Evidence of tight linkage could be used as support for an etiological hypothesis associating that gene with the epilepsies. This approach has the advantage that for the disease of interest, linkage is by definition tight, and the specified cloned genes offer the best possibility of resolving genotype.

More specifically, the candidate gene approach asks: Does the disease phenotype cosegregate with a given cloned gene? Does the disease phenotype map to the same region as a candidate gene? The genes of proteins listed in Table 2 could produce a mutation for epilepsy since they have been linked pathophysiologically to epilepsies in experimental animals. If the protein suspected of causing genetic epilepsy in an experimental animal is also the cause of the human epilepsy, there may be enough homology between the animal and human proteins to use animal-derived DNA to extract the human DNA. A specific example is the GABA receptor, which interacts with the diazepines. The question is whether individuals within a family who have epilepsy also have the same allele for the GABA receptor gene. If the correlation were strong enough, it would implicate the particular gene in the disease for that family. Determination of the inheritance of a specific allele of the GABA receptor gene requires the ability to follow the gene in the family.

The candidate gene approach is very powerful in that it allows one to test directly whether a specific gene is involved in the development of epilepsy. It has the disadvantage that the gene one wants to test must be physically "in hand" (i.e., cloned) for its involvement to be tested. This means that the suspected gene must be identified, isolated, and synthesized, and its chromosomal location identified (see Table 2).

Suitability of Juvenile Myoclonic Epilepsy to Genetic Linkage Studies

Among the epilepsies classified by the International League Against Epilepsy, the more common generally afflict humans who are otherwise mentally and neurologically normal between seizures, have good to excellent responses to antiepileptic drugs, and, in specific instances, may have high remission rates after withdrawal of antiepileptic drugs (Delgado-Escueta et al. [12]). These epilepsies must be distinguished from the more progressive and debilitating epileptic encephalopathies, such as the Lennox-Gastaut syndrome, the heredofamilial myoclonic epilepsies of Hartung [30], Hunt [33], Koskiniemi et al. [42], Lafora and Glueck [43], Lundborg [46], Unverricht [87], and Zeman et al. [97], and myoclonic epilepsies with structural brain lesions, neuronal storage (King [40]; Zeman [97]), and mitochondrial myopathy (Askanas et al. [3]).

Epilepsies best suited for genetic linkage analysis are those most likely to be caused by a single mutant gene showing a Mendelian pattern of inheritance. Accordingly, the early childhood epilepsy syndrome of Doose, childhood absence epilepsy, juvenile myoclonic epilepsy (JME) of Janz, pure grand mal (tonic-clonic, clonic-tonic-clonic), benign rolandic epilepsies with centrotemporal spikes, and the progressive myoclonus epilepsies are ideal for genetic linkage studies. Because progressive myoclonic encephalopathies, pure grand mal and pure absence epilepsy of childhood are relatively rare in our patient population in Los Angeles, we have been studying families of patients with JME and childhood epilepsy syndromes with combinations of tonic-clonic, myoclonic, and absence seizures. These forms of epilepsy are available in our population bases and provide informative pedigrees for genetic linkage studies (Delgado-Escueta and Greenberg [11]).

JME was first described by Herpin in 1852 and Rabot in 1899, but the Janz school in Berlin (Janz and Christian [38]) and the Comprehensive Epilepsy Program in Los Angeles (Delgado-Escueta and Enrile-Bacsal [10]) have been mainly responsible for its identification as a distinct and separate syndrome. In Europe, JME is also known as impulsive petit mal of Janz or the Herpin-Rabot-Janz syndrome. As the syndrome is recognized more frequently in different parts of the world, its recorded incidence among all epilepsies has grown from 2.7% in 1957 to 5.4% in 1977 and 11.9% in 1984. Most frequently, the syndrome starts at 13–15 years of age, with grand mal or tonic-clonic convulsions and minor myoclonic jerks. When tonic-clonic seizures are absent at onset, the condition frequently remains undiagnosed as minor irregular jerks of shoulders and arms that are mistaken for nervousness. When myoclonic jerks alone herald the onset of the syndrome, they also begin most commonly at 15 years of age. In such instances, major convulsions generally appear 2–3 years later. A series of successive myoclonic jerks that evolves into a tonic-clonic convulsion can usually be elicited from the patients history. Various authors report seizures mainly (52–95%) in the morning hours after awakening, induced by lack of sleep or premature awakening, and aggravated by fatigue or alcohol. Between 10% and 37% of patients also have absence epilepsy which starts in late childhood or adolescence. Rapid 4–6 Hz polyspike-wave complexes characterize the interictal EEG in almost all untreated patients. Ten percent have the classical 3 Hz spike-wave sequences or polyspike-wave complexes mixed with the rapid 4–6 Hz polyspike-wave complexes. Some 25–39% of families have first- or second-degree relatives with epileptic seizures (Delgado-Escueta et al. [13]; Janz [37]).

Recent analyses of its electroclinical traits in probands show that the syndrome persists into the 6th and 7th decades of life regardless of treatment (Delgado-Escueta and Enrile-Bacsal [10]; Janz [36]; Janz et al. [39]). This persistence of electroclinical traits during most of the patient's lifetime explains its high recurrence rate (90%) on withdrawal of drug treatment.

a

b

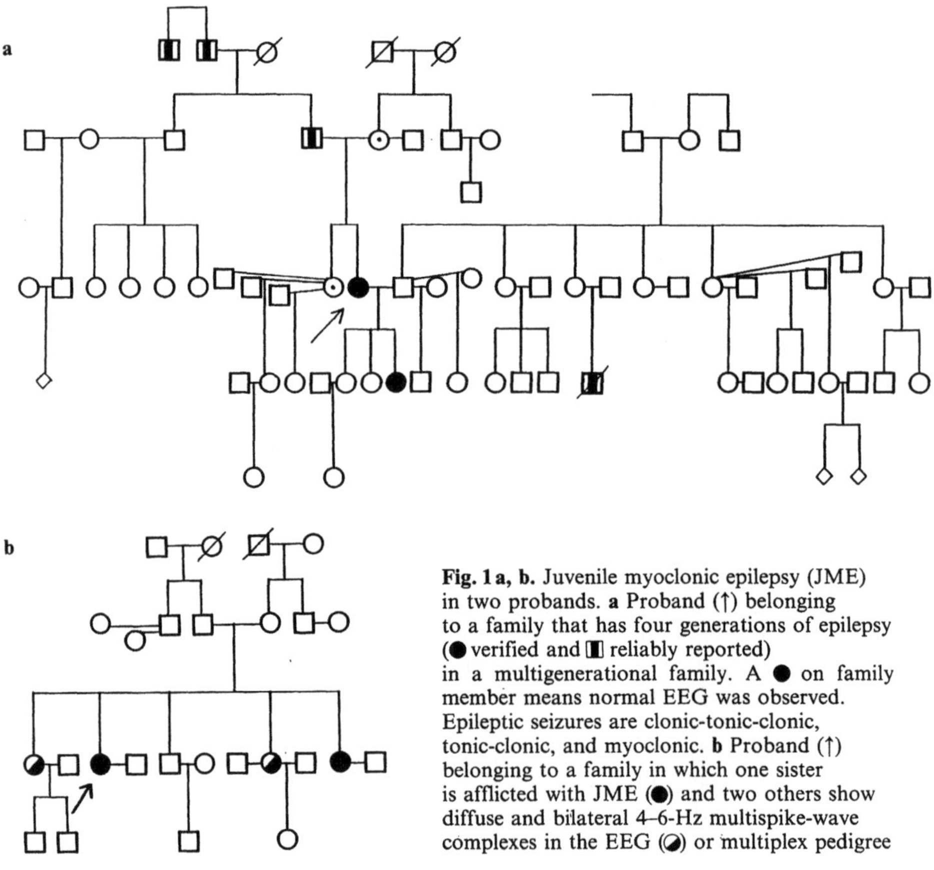

Fig. 1 a, b. Juvenile myoclonic epilepsy (JME) in two probands. **a** Proband (↑) belonging to a family that has four generations of epilepsy (● verified and ◨ reliably reported) in a multigenerational family. A ● on family member means normal EEG was observed. Epileptic seizures are clonic-tonic-clonic, tonic-clonic, and myoclonic. **b** Proband (↑) belonging to a family in which one sister is afflicted with JME (●) and two others show diffuse and bilateral 4–6-Hz multispike-wave complexes in the EEG (◕) or multiplex pedigree

Because the EEG trait may start as early as childhood and clinical seizures become evident at adolescence, and because both persist to late adulthood, it is possible to identify 3–4 generations of afflicted persons within a pedigree (Fig. 1). Most interestingly for genetic studies, the EEG trait of diffuse 3–6 Hz multispike-wave complexes is also inherited by asymptomatic siblings and not only by afflicted family members (Fig. 2). Because of this, we are able to identify more family members who carry the genes related to the expression of JME. Interestingly, we have also observed nonspecific but probably genetically determined paroxysmal abnormalities in parents and siblings of patients. These EEG traits consist

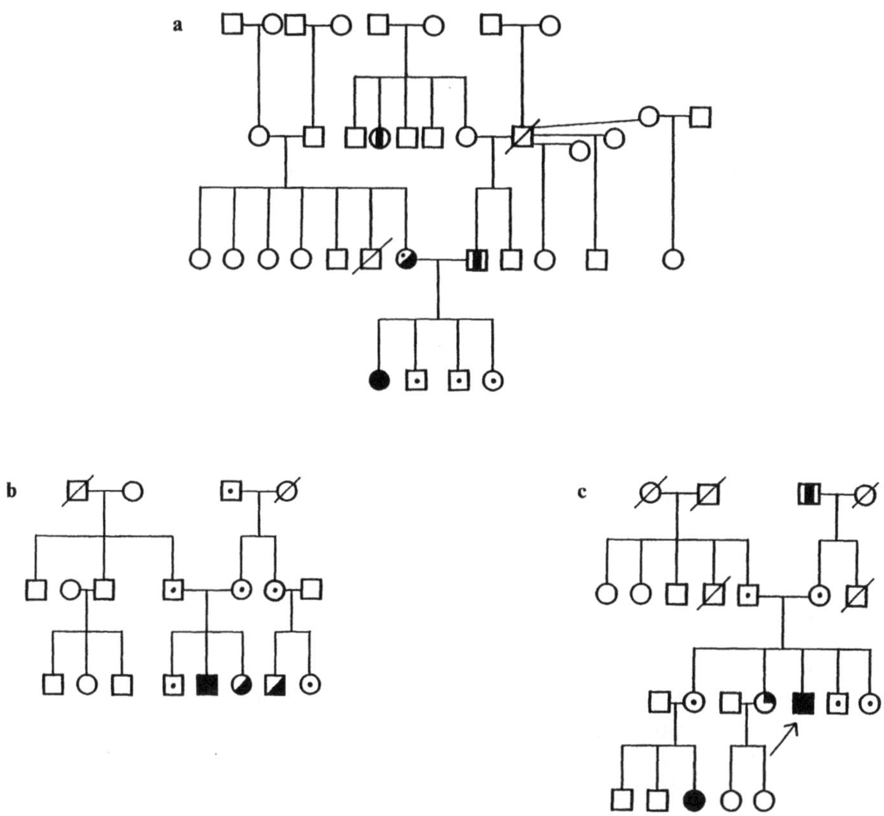

Fig. 2a–c. Juvenile myoclonic epilepsy in three probands. **a** Proband (↑ ●) whose pedigree is multigenerational by virtue of paroxysmal 4–7-Hz sharp waves and spikes in the mother (◕). Interestingly, the father and great aunt are reliably reported to have myoclonic jerks. **b** Proband (↑■) has a sister whose EEG shows diffuse bilateral 3–6-Hz multispike-wave complexes (◕). The mother's sister had normal EEG (⊙) but her son (proband's first-degree cousin) also had diffuse bilateral 3–6-Hz multispike-wave complexes. **c** Proband (↑■) has a sister whose EEG showed repetitive focal spikes (◔) and another sister with a normal EEG but with an afflicted daughter (●) – the proband's niece. The proband's mother also has a normal EEG but the maternal grandfather is reliably reported to have clonic-tonic-clonic and myoclonic seizures

of diffuse paroxysmal 3–6 Hz slow waves mixed with spike and sharp waves and/or diffuse paroxysmal 4–7 Hz waves (the paroxysmal theta waves of Doose and Gundel [15]). Doose and Gundel report that the presence of these nonspecific EEG abnormalities in parents increases the likelihood of their having symptomatic offspring, indicating that they are part of the total phenotype of JME. The frequency and ready availability of JME pedigrees, the presence of multiplex and multigenerational families with specific and nonspecific genetically determined EEG traits, the persistence of EEG and clinical traits during the patient's lifetime, and the relative seriousness of the grand mal and myoclonic epileptic attacks convinced us to use JME for genetic linkage studies.

Suitability of Idiopathic Generalized Epilepsies of Early Childhood to Genetic Linkage Studies

Severe epilepsies in early childhood (2–5 years of age) characterized by atypical absence drop attacks, tonic and tonic-clonic seizures associated with mental retardation, and an interictal irregular slow spike-wave EEG pattern (petit mal variant) are commonly called the Lennox-Gastaut syndrome. This syndrome is commonly differentiated from the less frequent primary generalized myoclonic-astatic epilepsy described by Doose et al. [18] and from other forms of generalized epilepsy of childhood (combined absence, tonic-clonic, myoclonic, and photoconvulsive seizures) where genetic predisposition plays a primary role. These latter epilepsies start in 1- to 5-year-old children with normal intelligence. The syndrome described by Doose affects boys three times more often than girls and is characterized by myoclonic, atonic, absence, and tonic-clonic seizures. Similar forms of seizure start at 5–10 years, shows no sex predisposition, but may be characterized by photosensitivity or self-induced absence attacks. All these generalized epilepsies of childhood show bilaterally synchronous irregular 2–3 Hz and 4–6 Hz multispike and wave complexes in the interictal EEG. Most of these syndromes respond well to valproic acid. By contrast, only a third of the secondary generalized myoclonic-astatic epilepsies with mental retardation which form the main group of the Lennox-Gastaut syndrome – a syndrome notoriously difficult to treat-respond to valproic acid, and then only partly.

In Lennox-Gestaut syndrome, children are affected at the age of 1–7 years and, with few exceptions, are severely mentally retarded. This condition is associated with the following: perinatal ischemic-hypoxic encephalopathy; intracranial hemorrhage; generalized, local, or unilateral cerebral atrophy; Toxoplasma and cytomegalovirus infections; tuberous sclerosis; phenylketonuria; nonketotic hyperglycinemia; and rare neurometabolic inherited diseases. Unlike in the genetically determined early childhood epilepsies, tonic seizures are more common in Lennox-Gastaut syndrome and appear with complex partial seizures, myoclonic, and drop seizures. The EEG shows the slow (<2 Hz) variety of spike/slow-wave complexes, multifocal spikes, runs of rapid spikes, and sometimes, hypsarrhythmia.

Often Lennox-Gastaut syndrome is preceded by infantile spasms, arrest of psychomotor development, and hypsarrhythmia. The latter triad is also called

West syndrome. The etiological factors responsible for Lennox-Gastaut syndrome overlap with those for West syndrome. A more fruitful approach toward both infantile spasms and Lennox-Gastaut syndrome would be to search for potentially reversible causes, institute early treatment, and hope for prevention of mental retardation. Excellent response has been reported on early treatment of West syndrome with adrenocorticotrophic hormone (ACTH) but, unfortunately, mental and motor disabilities do not always improve when infantile spasms stop. Symptomatic relief in both West and Lennox-Gastaut syndromes may be brought about in a fourth of the patients by treatment with valproic acid or clonazepam.

Clues: Which Genes to Look At

In the last 5 years, we have assembled family data on 20 probands and their families, which included 30 genetic markers and EEG data on over 100 family members. Thus far, on the basis of segregation analysis, we have tested a fully reduced penetrant recessive mode, a recessive mode with reduced penetrance, and a dominant mode with reduced penetrance as the modes of inheritance of JME. JME may well be a heterogenous disorder. For early childhood generalized epilepsies that are clearly distinct from Lennox-Gastaut syndrome, heterogeneity is also obvious, and autosomal dominant transmission may be present in some families.

In approaching these early childhood and adolescent epilepsy syndromes, we have utilized clues provided by dominantly inherited diseases associated with epilepsy and previous reports on HLA typing in absence epilepsies. These clues provide reasons for concentrating on genetic markers of chromosome 1 and chromosome 6. Classic Charcot-Marie-Tooth (CMT) hereditary neuropathy with autosomal dominant inheritance is linked to the Duffy blood group locus known to be on the long arm of chromosome 1 (Bird et al. [4]; Fig. 3). Rarely, grand mal and myoclonic epilepsy have been found in families of CMT patients. Lymphoblast and fibroblast cell lines should thus be collected from patients and their families who have both Charcot-Marie-Tooth disease and JME. Because the Duffy marker spans p22 and q25 and probably measures around 10–15 cM, we can theoretically use 26 markers, 20 cloned genes, and 6 cloned arbitrary segments mapped between p22 and q25. Moreover, the genes for the nerve growth factor and amylase, both of which reside within this location, are available as markers. Projects which screen recombinant libraries of purified chromosome 1 would also be extremely helpful. Purified chromosome preparations have been made using flow microfluorometry procedures and especially dual channel flow cytometry. These libraries should facilitate screening with flanker markers, and the use of these highly polymorphic markers should help accelerate the process of isolating possible epilepsy sites in chromosome 1.

Dominantly inherited spinocerebellar ataxia akin to Marie's ataxia has been linked to the HLA (human leucocyte antigen) locus on chromosome 6 (Jackson et al. [35]). This is a second clue to a possible site or sites for adolescent and childhood epilepsy syndromes because epilepsy has also been found in association with this form of hereditary ataxia. Association of HLA with epilepsies provides fur-

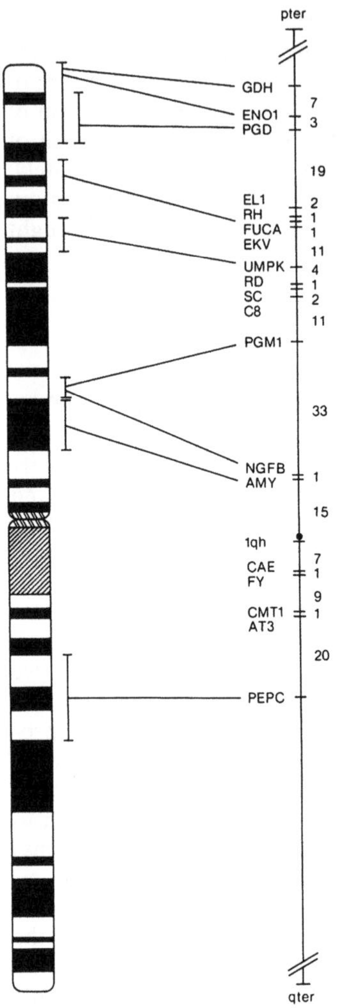

Fig. 3. The male genetic map of chromosome 1 with some points on the physical map shown for comparison. Distance in centimorgans. Note position of FY marker (Duffy) linked with Charcot-Marie-Tooth Syndrome. (Reproduced with permission from Human Gene Mapping 8, Cytogenetics and Cell Genetics, vol 40, 1985, p 95)

ther proof that an epilepsy site may be present in chromosome 6 (Table 3). Two independent reports (Rivas [71]; Fichsel and Kessler [22]) suggest that pure absence epilepsy is associated with alleles of the major histocompatibility complex or HLA on chromosome p6. These investigators found an increased incidence of A1-B8 haplotype in probands with absence epilepsy. Eeg-Olofsson et al. [21], however, found the opposite results. A decreased incidence of A1-B8 haplotype was observed in 16 probands with absence and 21 probands with rolandic epilepsy (see Table 3). Monaghan et al. [53] investigated the genetic association of the HLA haplotypes with cryptogenic myoclonic epilepsy in 29 probands and found no significant association.

Although the above reports on association between HLA haplotypes and epilepsy give conflicting results, it is possible that differences may be accounted for

Table 3. HLA and epilepsies

Type of Epilepsy	Number of families or probands	HLA	Author
Absence	25	Increased association with A1–B8	Fichsel and Kessler (1980)
Absence	42	Increased association with A1–B8	Rivas (1983)
Absence	16	Decreased incidence of A1–B8 haplotype	Eeg-Olofson et al. (1982)
Rolandic	21	Decreased incidence of A1–B8 haplotype	Eeg-Olofson et al. (1982)
Astatic myoclonic	19	No association	Howitz and Platz (1978)
Infantile spasms	40	Increased association with HLA–B7	Smeraldi et al. (1975)

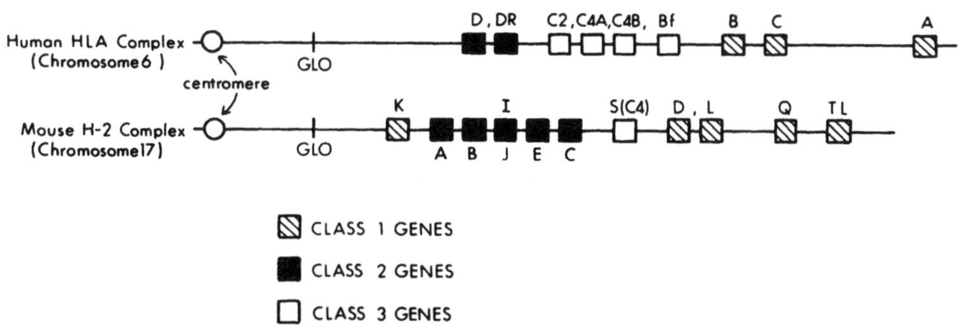

Fig. 4. Schematic diagram of the homologous functional classes of MHC genes in humans and mice. (Reproduced with permission from Stanburg et al. 1983)

by the heterogeneous nature of the epilepsies studied, the incomplete analysis of unexpanded families, and the failure of these studies to use the EEG "diffuse multispike-wave complex" as a genetic trait in linkage analysis. These early reports provide important clues which are worth pursuing. Thus, at present we are seeking both association and linkage between adolescent and childhood epilepsy syndromes and nearly 100 known HLA-A, B, C, and DR specificities (Laman and Olaisen [44]).

Figure 4 is a schematic diagram of the homologous functional classes of the HLA supergene (Fischer [23]) in humans and mice. The array of closely linked gene loci which evolved together to function as a unit in chromosome 6 in humans (Amos and Kostyu [2]) and in chromosome 17 in mice (Klein [41]) is illustrated. Interestingly, two class-1 proteins in mice have been identified as differentiation antigens on T cells and on some leukemia cells. A series of semi-lethal genes called the T/t complex regulates embryonic differentiation and effectively suppresses recombination along the chromosome carrying H-2. In these same loci, linkage has been described to audiogenic seizures (Seyfried et al. [75]) and the quaker mutant with seizures and ataxia. In humans a similar phenomenon may exist; a locus regulating spinal development has been mapped to the sixth chromosome (Amos and Kostyu [2]). In this regard, HLA linkage of spinocerebellar ataxia or olivopontocerebellar ataxia assumes significance (see Fig. 4).

Most recently, we have encountered the association of an early childhood epilepsy syndrome (absence, myoclonic, drop attacks and tonic seizures, clonic-tonic-clonic seizures) and the classical form of adrenogenital syndrome produced by a deficiency of 21-hydroxylase. 21-Hydroxylase is an enzyme required for complete adrenal steroidegenesis from cholesterol, the parent substance (Bongiovanni [5]). Excessive adrenocorticotrophic hormone production and the accumulation of cortisol precursors, particularly 17-OH progesterone, result, and secretion of abnormal quantities of androgens causes virilization prenatally or postnatally. 21-Hydroxylase deficiency is inherited as an autosomal recessive trait. During the seventh Los Angeles Conference on Human Gene Mapping, the gene for 21-hydroxylase was placed within the HLA region between HLA-B and HLA-D near properdin, or Factor B or BF (Dupont et al. [20]; Allen [1]). White et al. [91, 92] recently showed that 21-OH deficiency may result from the deletion of a specific cytochrome P_{450} gene. These authors also located two genes that encode 21-OH, 21-OHA and 21-OHB, located near the 3′ end of each of two C4 loci. The early childhood epilepsy syndrome associated with 21-OHA in our proband may be located within the same HLA class III region, where deletions and insertions appear to be frequent. Appropriate studies to document linkage are now in progress.

References

1. Allen FH Jr (1974) Linkage of HLA and GBG. Vox Sang 27:383–384
2. Amos DB, Kostyu DD (1980) HLA – a central immunological agency of man. Adv Hum Genet 10:137
3. Askanas V, Engel WK, Britton DE, Adornato BT, Eiben RM (1978) Reincarnation in cultured muscle of mitochondrial abnormalities. Two patients with epilepsy and lactic acidosis. Arch Neurol 35:801–809
4. Bird TD, Ott J, Giblett ER (1982) Evidence for linkage of Charcot-Marie-Tooth neuropathy to the Duffy locus on chromosome 1. Am J Hum Genet 34:388–394
5. Bongiovanni AM (1978) Congenital adrenal hyperplasia and related conditions. In Stanbury JB, Wyngaarden JB, Fredrickson DS (eds) The metabolic basis of inherited disease. McGraw-Hill, New York, p 868
6. Botstein D, White RL, Skolnick M, Davis RW (1980) Construction of a genetic linkage map in man using restriction fragment length polymorphisms. Am J Hum Genet 32:314–331
7. Caskey CT, White RI (eds) (1983) Banbury report 14: Recombinant DNA applications to human disease. Cold Spring Harbor, NY, Cold Spring Harbor Laboratory
8. Collins FS, Weissman SM (1984) Directional cloning of DNA fragments at a large distance from an initial probe: a circulation method. Proc Natl Acad Sci Genet USA 81:6812–6816
9. Conneally PM, Rivas MC (1980) Linkage analysis in man Adv Hum Genet 10:209–266
10. Delgado-Escueta AV, Enrile-Bacsal F (1984) Juvenile myoclonic epilepsy of Janz. Neurology (NY) 34:285–294
11. Delgado-Escueta AV, Greenberg D (1984) The search for epilepsies ideal for clinical and molecular genetic studies. Ann Neurol 16 (suppl) 2:1–11

12. Delgado-Escueta AV, Treiman DM, Walsh GO (1983) The treatable epilepsies. N Engl J Med 308:1508–1514 and 1576–1584
13. Delgado-Escueta AV, White R, Greenberg DA, Treiman LJ (1986) Looking for epilepsy genes: clinical and molecular genetic studies. In: Delgado-Escueta AV, Ward AA Jr, Woodbury DM, Porter RJ (eds) Advances in neurology, vol 44. New York, pp 77–95
14. DeLorenzo RJ (1986) A molecular approach to the calcium signal in brain: Relationship to synaptic modulation and seizure discharge. In: Delgado-Escueta AV, Ward AA Jr, Woodbury DM, Porter RJ (eds) Advances in neurology, vol 44. New York, pp 435–465
15. Doose H, Gundel A (1982) 4 to 7 CPS rhythms in the childhood EEG. In: Anderson VE, Hauser WA, Penry JK, Sing CF (eds) Genetic basis of the epilepsies. Raven, New York, pp 83–93
16. Doose H, Scheffner D (1982) Zur Therapie und Prognose der Absencen. Med Welt, pp 1763–1767
17. Doose H, Gerken H, Hien-Völpel KF, Völzke E (1969) Genetics of photosensitive epilepsy. Neuropaediatrie 1:56–73
18. Doose H, Gerken H, Leonhardt R, Völzke E, Völz C (1970) Centrencephalic myoclonic-astatic petit mal. Neuropädiatrie 2:59–78
19. Doose H, Gerken H, Horstmann T, Völzke E (1973) Genetic factors in spike wave absences. Epilepsia 14:57–75
20. Dupont B, Smithwick EM, Oberfield SE, Lee TD, Levine LS (1977) Close genetic linkage between HLA and congenital adrenal hyperplasia (21-hydroxylase deficiency). Lancet II:1309–1312
21. Eeg-Olofsson O, Safwenberg J, Wigertz A (1982) HLA and epilepsy: an investigation of different types of epilepsy in children and their families. Epilepsia 23:27–34
22. Fichsel H, Kessler M (1980) Immunogenetics of 3/s-SW absence epilepsy: frequency of HLA antigeness and haplotypes in patients and relatives. In: Canger R, Angeleri F, Penry JK (eds) Advances in epileptology (11th epilepsy international symposium). Raven, New York, pp 475–477
23. Fischer SG, Lerman LS (1983) DNA fragments differing by single base-pair substitutions are separated in denaturing gradient gels: correspondence with melting theory. Proc Natl Acad Sci USA 80(6):1579–1583
24. Gedda L, Tatarelli R (1971) Essential isochronic epilepsy in MZ twin pairs. Acta Genet Med 20:380–383
25. Grisar T, Franck G, Delgado-Escueta AV (1983) Glial contribution to seizures: K^+ activation of (Na^+K^+)-ATPase in bulk isolated glial cells and synaptosomes of epileptogenic cortex. Brain Res 261:75–85
26. Gusella JF, Wexler NS, Conneally PM et al. (1983) A polymorphic DNA marker genetically linked to Huntington's disease. Nature 306:234–238
27. Gusella JF, Tanzi RE, Anderson MA, Hobbs W, Gibbons K, Raschtchian R, Gilliam TC, Wallace M, Wexler NS, Conneally PM (1984) DNA markers for nervous system disease. Science 225:1320–1326
28. Haldane JBS, Smith CAB (1974) A new estimate of linkage between the genes for color blindess and haemophilia in man. Ann Engen 14:10–31
29. Harper PS, Rivas ML, Bias WB, Hutchinson JR, Dyken PR, McKusick VA (1972) Genetic linkage confirmed between the locus for myotonic dystrophy and the ABH secretion and Lutheran blood group loci. Am J Hum Genet 24:310
30. Hartung E (1920) Zwei Fälle von Paramyoclonus multiplex mit Epilepsie. Z Gesamte Neurol Psychiatr 56:151–153
31. Herpin TH (1852) Du pronostic et traitement curatif de l'épilepsie. Ouvrage couronné par l'institut de France en 1850, 2 p 1, 622 pp. Paris, Baillière
32. Hodge SE, Anderson CE, Neiswanger K et al. (1983) The search for heterogeneity in insulin dependent diabetes mellitus (IDDM): linkage studies, two locus models, and genetic heterogeneity. Am J Hum Genet 35:1139–1155
33. Hunt JR (1921) Dyssynergia cerebellaris myoclonica – Primary atrophy of the dentate system: a contribution to the pathology and symptomatology of the cerebellum. Brain 44:490–538

34. Iadorola MJ, Gale K (1982) Substantia nigra: site of anticonvulsant activity mediated by γ-aminobutyric acid. Science 218:1237–1240
35. Jackson JF, Currier RD, Terasaki PI, Morton NE (1977) Spinocerebellar ataxia and HLA linkage. N Engl J Med 296:1138
36. Janz D (1982) In tema di remissione e di ricomparsa di crisi durante e dopo il trattamento farmacologico dell'epilessia. Boll Lega Ital Epil 39:95–100
37. Janz D (1985) Epilepsy with impulsive petit mal (Juvenile myoclonic epilepsy). Acta Neurol Scand 72:449–459
38. Janz D, Christian W (1957) Impulsiv-petit mal. Dtsch Z Nervenheilk 19:155–182
39. Janz D, Kern A, Mössinger HJ, Puhlmann HU (1982) Rückfallprognose während und nach Reduktion der Medikamente bei Epilepsiebehandlung. In: Remschmidt H, Rentz R, Jungmann J (eds) Epilepsie 1981. Thieme, Stuttgart, pp 311–318
40. King JO (1975) Progressive myoclonic epilepsy due to Gaucher's disease in an adult. J Neurol Neurosurg Psychiatry 38:849–854
41. Klein J (1979) The major histocompatibility complex of the mouse. Science 203:516
42. Koskiniemi M, Toivakka E, Donner M (1974) Progressive myoclonus epilepsy, electroencephalographic findings. Acta Neurol Scand 50:333–359
43. Lafora GR, Glueck B (1911) Contributions to the histopathology and pathogenesis of myoclonic epilepsy. Bull Gov Hosp Insane 3:96
44. Lamman LU, Olaisen B (1985) Report of the committee on the genetic constitution of chromosome six. Cytogenet Cell Genet 31:129–155
45. Lennox WG, Lennox MA (1960) Epilepsy and related disorders. Little Brown, Boston
46. Lundborg H (1912) Der Erbgang der progressiven Myoklonusepilepsie. Z Gesamte Neurol Psychiatr 9:353–358
47. Matthes A (1969) Genetic studies in epilepsy. In: Gastaut H, Jasper H, Bancaud J, Waltregny A (eds) The physiopathogenesis of the epilepsies. Thomas, Springfield, pp 26–30
48. Matthes A, Weber H (1968) Klinische und elektroenzephalographische Familienuntersuchungen bei Pyknolepsien. Dtsch Med Wochenschr 93:429–435
49. McKusick VA (1983) Mendelian inheritance in man. In: Catalogs of autosomal dominant, autosomal recessive and X-linked phenotypes, 5th edn. John Hopkins University Press, Baltimore
50. McKusick VA (1986) Mapping the human genome: status, interpretation and prospects. 7th International Congress of Human Genetics, Berlin, abstracts vol 1, no 12
51. Metrakos K, Metrakos JD (1961) Genetics of convulsive disorders. II. Genetic and electroencephalographic studies in centrencephalic epilepsy. Neurology (Minn) 11:474–483
52. Mohr J (1954) A study of linkage in man. Munksgaard, Copenhagen
53. Monaghan HP, O'Sullivan M, O'Donohoe NV (1982) HLA antigens and cryptogenic myoclonic epilepsy. J Med Sci 151(6):188–189
54. Morton ME (1962) Segregation and linkage. In: Burdette (ed) Methodology in human genetics. Holden Day, San Francisco, pp 17–52
55. Narahashi T (1986) Modulators acting on sodium and calcium channels: Patch clamp analysis. Delgado-Escueta AV, Ward AA Jr, Woodbury DM, Porter RJ (eds) Advances in neurology, vol 44. Raven, New York, pp 211–225
56. Noebels JL (1979) Analysis of inherited epilepsy using single locus mutations in mice. Fed Proc 38:2405–2410
57. Noebels JL (1982) Defined gene models of the inherited epilepsies. In: Anderson VE, Hauser WA, Penry JK, Sing CF. Genetic basis of the epilepsies. New York, pp 211–224
58. Olsen RW, Snowmen AM, Lee R, Lomax P, Wamsley JK (1984) Role of the γ-aminobutyric acid receptor/ionophore complex in seizure disorders. Ann Neurol 16(S):90–95
59. Ott J (1977) Counting methods (EM algorithm) in human pedigree analysis. Ann Hum Genet 40:443–454
60. Ounsted C (1952) The factor of inheritance in convulsive disorders in childhood. Proc Soc Med 45:865–868
61. Overweg J, Rowan AJ, Binnie CD, Nagelkerke NJD, Costing J (1981) Prediction of seizure recurrence after withdrawal of antiepileptic drugs. In: Dam M, Gram L, Penry JK (eds) Advances in epileptology: 12th epilepsy international symposium. Raven, New York, pp 503–508

62. Pedersen HE, Krogh E (1970) Decentraliseret behandling og kontrol af patienter med epilepsi. Nord Med 83:689–694
63. Penry JK, Porter R, Dreifuss FE (1975) Simultaneous recordings of absence seizures with videotape and EEG. Brain 98:427–440
64. Pericak-Vance MA, Conneally PM, Merritt AD, Roos R, Vance JM, Yu PL, Norton JA, Angel JP (1979) In: Chase TMN, Wexler NS, Barbeen A (eds) Advances in neurology. Raven, New York, p 59
65. Pericak-Vance MA, Stajich JM, Conneally PM, Vance J, Herbstreith MH, Roses AD (1983) Genetic linkage analysis of myotonic dystrophy with the complement component 3 (C3), secretor (Se), and Lewis (Le) loci on chromosome 19. Program abstracts, 7th International Human Gene Mapping Workshop, University of California at Los Angeles, 21–26 Aug 1983
66. Phillips JA, Hjelle BL, Seeburg PH, Zachmann M (1981) Molecular basis for familial isolated growth hormone deficiency. Proc Natl Acad Sci USA 78:6372–6375
67. Rabot M (1899) De la myoclonie épileptique. Thesis, Paris
68. Rapport RL II, Harris AB, Friel PN, Ojemann GA (1975) Human epileptic brain $Na^{+}K^{+}$ -ATPase activity and phenytoin concentrations. Arch Neurol 32:549–554
69. Rigby PW, Dieckmann M, Rhodes C, Berg P (1977) Labeling deoxyribonucleic acid to high specific activity in vitro by nick translation with DNA polymerase I. J Mol Biol 113(1):237–251
70. Rimoin DL, Metrakos JD (1964) The genetics of convulsive disorders in the families of hemiplegics. Proc 2nd Int Congr Hum Genet 3:1655–1658
71. Rivas ML (1983) Genetic analysis of petit mal epilepsy I. Evaluation of HLA, blood groups, serum proteins, and red cell enzymes. Epilepsia 24:115
72. Roses AD, Pericak-Vance MA, Yamaoka LH (1983) Recombinant DNA strategies in genetic neurological diseases. In: Austin L, Jeffrey PL (eds) Molecular aspects of neurological diseases. Academic, Sydney, pp 3–16
73. Sarfarazi M, Ball S, O'Brien T, Davies K, Shaw D, Harper PS (1983) Myotonic dystrophy and markers on chromosome 19. Program abstracts, 7th International Human Gene Mapping Workshop, University of California at Los Angeles, 21–26 Aug 1983
74. Seyfried TN (1982) Developmental genetics of audiogenic seizure susceptibility in mice. In: Anderson VE, Hauser WA, Penry JK, Sing CF (eds) Genetic basis of the epilepsies. Raven, New York, pp 199–210
75. Seyfried TN, Glaser GH, Yu RK, Palayoor ST (1986) Inherited convulsive disorders in mice. In: Delgado-Escueta AV, Ward AA Jr, Woodbury DM, Porter RJ (eds) Advances in neurology, vol 44. Raven, New York, pp 115–135
76. Shows TB, Sakaguchi AY, Naylor SL (1982) Mapping the human genome, cloned genes, DNA polymorphisms and inherited disease. Adv Hum Genet 12:341–353
77. Shows TB, McAlpine PV, Miller RL (1983) The 1983 catalogue of mapped human genetic markers and report of the nomenclature committee. Cytogenet Cell Genet 37:340–393
78. Skolnick MH, White R (1982) Strategies for detecting and characterizing restriction fragment length polymorphisms (RFLPs) Cytogenet Cell Genet 32:58–67
79. Southern EM (1975) Detection of specific sequences among DNA fragments separated by gel electrophoresis. J Mol Biol 98:503–517
80. Stanburg J, Wyngaarden JB, Fredrickson DS, Goldstein JL, Brown MS (eds) (1983) Metabolic basis of inherited diseases. McGraw-Hill, New York, chap 3, p 79
81. Terasaki PI (ed) (1980) Histocompatibility testing. UCLA tissue typing laboratory 1980
82. Tower DB (1965) Problems associated with studies of electrolyte metabolism in normal and epileptogenic cerebral cortex. Epilepsia 6:183
83. Tsuboi T (1980) Genetic aspects of epilepsy. Folia Psychiatr Neurol Jpn 34:215–225
84. Tsuboi T, Christian W (1973) On the genetics of primary generalized epilepsy with sporadic myoclonias of the impulsive petit mal type: A clinical and electroencephalographic study of 399 probands. Humangenetik 19:155–182
85. Tsuboi T, Endo S (1977) Incidence of seizures and EEG abnormalities among offspring of epileptic patients. Hum Genet 36:173–189
86. Tudor I, Milea S, Bicescu E, Ivana D (1973) Catamnestic study of childhood epilepsy. Rev Roum Neurol 10:341–352

87. Unverricht H (1891) Die Myoklonie. Deuticke, Leipzig
88. Vogel F, Motulsky AG (1979) Human genetics: Problems and approaches. Springer, Berlin Heidelberg New York
89. Ward RH (1982) Genetics and epidemiology: a fruitful interface for the study of epilepsy. In: Anderson VE, Hauser WA, Penry JK, Sing CF (eds) Genetic basis of the epilepsies. Raven, New York, pp 317–332
90. Weinstock GM, Rhys C, Berman ML, Hampar B, Jackson D, Silhary TJ, Weisemann J, Zweig M (1983) Open reading frame expression vectors: a general method for antigen production in Escherichia coli using protein fusions to beta-galactosidase. Proc Natl Acad Sci USA 80(14):4432–4436
91. White PC, New MI, Dupont B (1984) HLA linked congenital adrenal hyperplasia results from defective gene encoding a cytochrome P-450 specific for 21-hydroxylation. Proc Natl Acad Sci USA 81:7505–7509
92. White PC, Grossberger D, Onufer B, Chaplin D, New MI, Dupont B, Strominger JL (1985) Two genes encoding steroid 21-hydroxylase are located near the genes encoding the fourth component of complement in man. Proc Natl Acad Sci USA 82:1089–1093
93. White R (1984) Looking for epilepsy genes. Ann Neurol 16 [Suppl] 2:12–17
94. Wyman AR, White R (1980) A highly polymorphic locus in human DNA. Proc Natl Acad Sci USA 77:6754–6758
95. Zatz M, Vianna-Morgante AM, Campos P, Diament AJ (1981) Translocation (X:6) in a female with Duchenne muscular dystrophy: Implications for the localization of the DMD locus. J Med Genet 19:442
96. Zeman W (1976) The neuronal ceroid-lipo fuscinoses. In: Zimmerman HM (ed) Progress in neuropathology, vol 3. Grune and Stratton, Orlando, pp 203–223
97. Zeman W, Donahue S, Dyken P, Green J (1970) The neuronal ceroidlipofuscinoses (Batten-Vogt syndrome). In: Vinken PJ, Bruyn GW (eds) Handbook of neurology, vol 10. North-Holland, Amsterdam, pp 588–679

Closing Remarks

V. E. Anderson [1]

The successful completion of this workshop owes much to Dieter Janz for suggesting the idea early in 1985, to Karl Sperling for announcing it as a satellite meeting of the 7th International Congress of Human Genetics, and to Gertrud Beck-Mannagetta for planning and coordinating the scientific presentations and arrangements. The effect has been to focus the attention of human geneticists on epilepsy, to provide epileptologists with exposure to advances in human genetics, and to speed up the analysis and interpretation of data combining these two important areas of research.

The papers presented in this workshop give evidence of significant progress since July of 1980, when many of the same participants met in Minnesota. The level of effective conversation has improved markedly among the specialists involved in the multidisciplinary research effort – neurologists, geneticists, epidemiologists, and biochemists. New studies have been initiated, and pre-existing ones have been enlarged and strengthened as the result of collaborative efforts. Even the discussion of the papers was better informed and more constructive. At the conclusion we were left with a clearer view of the research agenda for the next few years.

A central issue is still the classification of seizures and seizure syndromes. Much recent effort has gone into the revision of taxonomic schemes in order to improve the clinical care of epilepsy patients. In genetic studies, however, we must consider the changes in seizure type and EEG pattern that can take place over an individual's lifetime. We do not yet understand how much variability is possible in the expression of a given syndrome, and thus cannot determine with reasonable certainty whether an affected relative's seizures represent the same syndrome found in the proband or a different condition. Our goal is to develop a taxonomy that does not depend on age, severity, or family history, since those variables should be used to *study* a syndrome, not to *define* it. The papers in this workshop represent an essential intermediate step toward that final goal.

We also recognize the importance of maintaining a variety of research strategies. The most expensive, yet absolutely essential, approach involves longitudinal studies which follow subjects throughout the major period of risk for seizures. Studies of offspring are longitudinal in a different sense because they involve an entire generation's time span. Reports from a generation ago may provide a valuable baseline for both of these methods. For some questions we need representa-

[1] Department of Genetics and Cell Biology, Dight Laboratories, University of Minnesota, 400 Church Street S.E., Minneapolis, MN 55455, USA.

Genetics of the Epilepsies
Beck-Mannagetta et al. (Eds.)

tive samples of populations, while for others it is much more efficient to select series of patients with a specific type of epilepsy. Interesting observations from any one study must be checked and verified in another setting, but the data must have been collected in a form that permits direct comparison. Thus, the patterns of collaboration fostered by workshops such as this become a part of a total research design.

The development of new research methods gives hope that answers may be found for some of the vexing problems in epilepsy research. Questions about etiology and treatment require new applications of existing biochemical methods and the design of new techniques. The detection of linkage between genetic markers and one of the seizure phenotypes will trigger efforts to map other seizure-related gene loci. The clinical variability in some seizure syndromes may turn out to involve the "microdeletion" of a varying number of closely linked genes to produce what have been termed "contiguous gene syndromes." Rapidly growing knowledge about the brain-specific expression of genes will generate new methods for analyzing brain structure and function. Finally, transgenic animal models of genetic diseases will be constructed first for simpler biochemical disorders, but eventually may be available for the study of seizures.

The papers in this volume thus provide excellent illustrations of research methods for the genetic analysis of seizures and epilepsy. They should be of interest to workers in clinical and experimental epileptology as well as to human geneticists. Taken together, they renew our hope that genetics will be a major contributor to a comprehensive and intergrated view of seizures and epilepsy.

Subject Index

H.-H. Frey, D. Janz, Berlin (Eds.)

Antiepileptic Drugs

1985. 54 figures. XXII, 867 pages. (Handbook of Experimental Pharmacology, Volume 74). Hard cover
ISBN 3-540-13108-6

"...this book will be the standard reference book on epileptic drugs not only for clinicians dealing with the problem of epilepsy but also for basic scientists investigating the effects of the drugs in experimental animals."

"...this book is going to be mandatory in a laboratory or clinic library where investigation of antiepileptic drugs is being carried out."

Archives internationales de Pharmacodynamie et de Therapie

Springer-Verlag
Berlin Heidelberg New York
London Paris
Tokyo Hong Kong

Springer

MIX
Papier aus verantwortungsvollen Quellen
Paper from responsible sources
FSC® C105338
FSC
www.fsc.org

If you have any concerns about our products,
you can contact us on
ProductSafety@springernature.com

In case Publisher is established outside the EU,
the EU authorized representative is:
Springer Nature Customer Service Center GmbH
Europaplatz 3, 69115 Heidelberg, Germany

Printed by Libri Plureos GmbH
in Hamburg, Germany